The Portable Personal Trainer

The Portable Personal Trainer

100 Ways to Energize Your Workouts and Bring Out the Athlete in You

ERIC HARR

Foreword by Nine-Time Olympic Medalist Dara Torres

Broadway Books
New York

BROADWAY

Broadway Books titles may be purchased for business or promotional use or for special sales. For information, please write to: Special Markets Department, Random House, Inc., 1540 Broadway, New York, NY 10036.

BROADWAY BOOKS and its logo, a letter B bisected on the diagonal, are trademarks of Broadway Books, a division of Random House, Inc.

Visit our website at www.broadwaybooks.com

Library of Congress Cataloging-in-Publication Data
Harr, Eric, 1971–
    The portable personal trainer : 100 ways to energize your workouts and bring out the athlete in you / Eric Harr.—1st ed.
        p. cm.
    1. Physical fitness. 2. Physical fitness—Psychological aspects. 3. Exercise. 4. Exercise—Psychological aspects. I. Title.
    GV481 .H2555 2001
    613.7'1—dc21   00-069792

FIRST EDITION

Designed by Ellen Cipriano

ISBN 0-7679-0641-1

01 02 03 04 05 10 9 8 7 6 5 4 3 2 1

For Mom and Dad.
And for the most passionate person I've ever met,
my lovely wife, Alexandra.

Acknowledgments

I would like to acknowledge my literary agent, Robert Preskill, and Jennifer Griffin for being the first people to believe in me in the publishing world. And my best friends:

Chris, Clarke, Joe, Oliver, Sharon, Walter, and Gramma.

The Portable Personal Trainer

Foreword

I first met Eric Harr on the peak of Mount Tamalpais in Marin County, California, as we shot the pilot of a new thirteen-part documentary series called *Building a Champion: The Inside Secrets of the World's Best Athletes*. In the series, Eric and I travel the globe, training with the best athletes in each culture. We want to learn what really makes them champions—the premise being that the secrets to true fitness reside in the hearts and heads of champion athletes the world over, not in quick-fix plans or new abdomen exercises. Eric conceived the series; in fact, it's based on many of the same principles as is this wonderful book.

A few words about Eric before I get to his book. The first things I noticed about Eric upon meeting him were his intensity and excitement. From what I've seen, his charisma is infectious, and he can inspire people to reach for new levels of achievement. I've been training competitively as a swimmer for over eighteen years, and I've never met anyone like him. He draws people's passions right to the surface, encouraging them to strive for goals they believed were out of reach.

Eric is also one of the best triathletes in the world. Even in the highest athletic circles, the triathlon event is known to be one of the most physically demanding sports. Here's a sport that requires you to perform at a world-class level in three distinctly different arenas. It takes an incredible amount of discipline, knowledge, and determination to succeed in this sport. Eric not only succeeded—he was the first rookie ever to be ranked in the world Top 10.

In *The Portable Personal Trainer,* Eric has distilled the wisdom of a triathlete and combined that with commonsense training tips. The result is a book like no other: a portable, inspirational guide to exercising (and living) to the fullest. And because he's the "real deal" himself, Eric has inside access to the secrets of the world's best athletes. What makes this book so special is that he breaks those high-level concepts into simple ideas and makes them apply to anyone's fitness program. He has encapsulated the best fitness advice from around the world in 100 simple strategies. This book is a unique treasure. I've read hundreds of fitness, diet, and motivational books—trust me on this.

What do I love most about this book? It's right on the money and it's just a whole lot of fun. I've trained with the best coaches, athletes, nutritionists, and mental coaches, and the best fitness advice I've learned is to exercise intelligently (instead of just as hard as you can) and to have fun. It's really that simple. Do these two things and you'll get more physical, mental, and spiritual fitness results than you can possibly imagine.

This remarkable book will show you how.

Dara Torres

Introduction

Nothing great was ever achieved without enthusiasm.
—RALPH WALDO EMERSON, WRITER (1803–1882)

Passion and performance. As a professional athlete in the world's most physically demanding sport, I've spent every waking minute of every day for the past seven years seeking to master these two words.

My career as a triathlete began in the Virgin Islands. It was a serendipitous discovery. I was biking to and from work in a law firm there and idly decided to do a local triathlon—despite being twenty pounds overweight and having zero background in cycling or running! As I began to train for this event, a passion ignited deep within me, and that passion fueled a new level of physical and mental performance, which further inspired me to exercise. This became a self-perpetuating cycle until, after four months, I was having so much fun exercising that everything I did had a new level of excitement. Winning that race improved my self-image, but the training process transformed my life.

The most fascinating part of this experience was the permanence of my new passion. It didn't wear off like the classic post-self-help seminar high. It didn't fade away like the excitement of reading an inspiring book or the buzz of setting New Year's resolutions. This was *my* body, and this passion came from the inside out. It came freely, it was permanent, and I owned the experience—nobody else could take credit for it. That was the best part. The new drive came from teaching my body and mind to perform by exercising smarter, not harder, and by focusing more on the pure enjoyment of exercise. I had ignited the "athlete" in me.

Today, triathlon is my career. It's not the most lucrative sport in the world, but I wouldn't give it up for the world. I am paid many times over in other ways. For me, triathlon is a tangible way to construct a more fulfilling and meaningful life, to keep my passion alive, to reach my true potential, to be fully happy. Isn't that what we all seek? You can achieve those things with something that is simple, fun, invigorating, and cost-free: exercise. Athletics elicit spirited emotion from people around the world, because we see the best parts of ourselves in action. We watch great athletes on television, not to worship their exceptional lives, but deep down to remind ourselves what is possible in our own.

But lately it seems that connection has broken down. In 2000 Americans spent $31.7 billion trying to lose weight, get fit, or boost their health, yet there are 52 million clinically obese people in this nation. We know more than we ever did before about health and fitness, but we're still not getting the results we want and deserve. This is due in part to an increasing reliance on others to solve our fitness and nutrition issues—when, in fact, *we* know more about our bodies than anyone else. It's time to pursue our goals from the inside out rather than the outside in.

The Portable Personal Trainer is designed to empower you with the tools and strategies that you need to rely on yourself for motivation and fitness results rather than paying someone else to help you. Where does the information in this book come from? Over the past seven years I recorded the most powerful lessons from tens of thousands of hours of my own training and generations of wisdom gleaned from the very best athletes in diverse cultures around the world—athletes with whom I've closely trained and competed. Through swimming with German triathletes in the U.S. Virgin Islands, mountain biking with Dutch national champions in Boulder, Colorado, and running with

Kenyans on an island off the coast of Morocco, I've become privy to their most prized secrets. I focused on how these people stay motivated and how they transform their passion into performance and that performance into even more passion for their sports and their lives. I watched these people *very closely* and chronicled their innermost wisdom. I've also read thousands of books and magazines related to health, fitness, and athletic performance in my quest to become the best athlete I can be.

You hold in your hands a collection of the best lessons from this experience, distilled into simple, palatable real-world strategies. By following them, you will learn how to gain the maximum physical and mental benefits from exercise and how to forge that new performance into a lifelong passion. Just as the world's best athletes do.

Champion athletes are the world's most reliable source of truth and wisdom on fitness. They have distilled years of experience into concise methods that *work*. They have tried and tested every tool, technique, and method to reach their goals, and their collective wisdom is a treasure trove of information that will excite and motivate us all.

The proven strategies in this book were forged not in books or in the laboratory, but on the roads and fields, in the pools and on the mountainsides, by the world's best athletes. Amazingly, anyone at any fitness level can use this information just the same as they do. In this book I will convey the most advanced fitness concepts from around the world in the simplest, most conversational way I can.

The first eight strategies presented here will create the foundation of your new fitness program. The rest of the tips will build on that foundation by showing you how to enjoy exercise more, get more from your workouts, stay motivated, and apply to your daily life the lessons learned during exercise. As I mention in tip #36, to build a rock-solid self-confidence, you must have a high degree of self-trust. So I ask that you incorporate one tip from this book into your life each day for four weeks. This is very potent advice that comes from the highest realm of the fitness world, and these tips will change your life in profound ways. Just give it four weeks and you'll see.

While implementing these tips, remember that world-class athletes are not a separate species from you. The NBA stars, the Kenyan runners, the Olympic swimmers, are ordinary people simply called to extraordinary circumstances. Many of these athletes are *not* genetically gifted—they perform mind-boggling feats because of their driving passion for their sports. That is the common thread of all great athletes around the globe: a genuine, rich passion for what they are doing. The love of their sport runs so deep that they will cycle for seven hours in the rain, run endless intervals, or swim tens of thousands of yards each day, every day, for years. Human passion is the most powerful force on earth. It fuels success in everything we do, from exercise to career to life. Tapping into that athlete in you can be a doorway to an empowering, enriching, passion-driven life.

Self-actualization, the joy of athletics, the thrill of better performance, and the hunger for passion are notions that are timeless and universal. They resonate in the hearts of us all, regardless of age, culture, or gender. They are the core concepts in this book that I hope will educate, inspire, and motivate you.

Exercise passion.

Eric Harr

1. Don't Just Dream Big, Dream Huge

~~~~~~

Twenty years from now you will be more disappointed by the things you didn't do than by the ones you did. So throw off the bowlines. Sail away from the safe harbor. Catch the trade winds in your sails. Explore. Dream!

—MARK TWAIN, WRITER (1835–1910)

How we've forgotten to dream! As we get older, our goals and our visions tend to grow smaller, more manageable, more "realistic." Our limiting beliefs are more confining than we realize. Nowhere is this truer than in our personal visions of health and exercise. We're constantly making excuses and concessions, and over time, some of us have resigned ourselves to a lower standard of fitness than we ever intended.

It's time to demand more from your body.

When I began training for triathlons seven years ago, I was overweight and had no background in cycling or running. Yet I decided that in one year I would be ranked in the world's top ten. People thought I was mad. I read and reread *Dave Scott's Triathlon Training* and followed his advice to the letter—so far as riding to work through torrential Caribbean downpours! Six months later I was ranked number six in the world.

You may not aspire to be a world-class athlete, but nevertheless you will benefit tremendously from this strategy. The first step to igniting your passion and opening the door to your boldest fitness goals is to set new goals that excite, inspire, and move you. Goals that reside "within your comfort zone" are unlikely to ignite your deepest passions. Setting new, passion-driven goals is the foundation of any successful fitness program.

~~~~~~

ACTION ITEM

Get outside. This exercise cannot be done indoors—to truly open up your mind to new fitness possibilities, oxygen must be coursing in your blood, your endorphins must be pumping, and your consciousness must be liberated. (In fact, I recommend you do most of the "action items" in this book while in motion, during exercise.)

Exercise at a nice, steady aerobic effort, and think about what you want from your body. When you complete your workout, pull out a fresh sheet of paper and write down your three boldest fitness goals. The trick here is to think *huge*. This is not about "thinking outside the box," it's about disregarding the box altogether. It doesn't mean you have to achieve those goals, but the sheer act of writing down new, lofty goals will begin the process of igniting your passion and will open the door to higher personal performance.

Now that your boldest goals are on paper, scale them back ever so slightly into the realm of realism. Olympic two-hundred-meter champion Michael Johnson's advice on goals is to make them *quantitative* and *time based* and *realistic*. Thinking huge first determines what's most important to you, what's really possible. This raises your own standards. You'll always have your eyes on that prize, and you just never know how close to those goals you may come.

Congratulations. What you just did is how champion athletes begin their quest toward world-record performances. They just dream absolutely huge.

2. Pinpoint Your Ends Motivations

~~~~~~

Every battle is won before it is fought.

—SUN TZU, FOURTH-CENTURY GENERAL, AUTHOR OF *THE ART OF WAR*

To enjoy long-term success in fitness, you need something to hold on to, something to motivate you, something to inspire you over the long term. If you can discover what that is, the battle of reaching your fitness goals "will have been won before it is fought."

Staying motivated is one of the most challenging elements of any fitness program. The first step is to clarify your deep-down motivations to work out. When you do this, you change your fitness destiny because you will be motivated to exercise more consistently and with more passion.

There are "means" motivations and "ends" motivations. Most people know their means motivations, which is why they often struggle to stay motivated to exercise. Top world-class athletes understand their ends motivations, which is why they *rarely* struggle to stay motivated. What do I mean?

"To lose ten pounds" is a means motivation. That is simply a *means* to an *end*. You don't really want to lose ten pounds. You want what losing ten pounds will give you, how it will make you feel. Will "I want to lose ten pounds" get you out the door every day, filled with passion and excitement for your workouts? Probably not. Your motivations must *really move you*. A better way to rephrase this motivation might be "Look, if I lose ten pounds, I will feel more passionate, I will look younger, and I will become a hell of a lot more attractive to the opposite sex!" Those ends motivations are more likely to inspire you to work out more often and with more passion.

~~~~~~

ACTION ITEM

Your long-term success in fitness relies on a true, rich understanding of your ends motivations. A written list of those motivations will keep your passion alive and reignite it when it fades. Sit alone in a quiet place and ask yourself why you want to achieve your bold new fitness goals. Be honest and emotionally charged as you write down those motivations, and post them where you can see them daily. When you're feeling uninspired, refer to the list. If the list does not motivate you, it's time to reassess what motivates you, and this may change often. Keep your list of ends motivations fresh, current, and passion driven, and it will provide you with a powerful wellspring of motivation to exercise.

3. Face Your Weaknesses

You cannot run away from a weakness; you must sometimes fight it out or perish; and if that be so, why not now and where you stand?

—Robert Louis Stevenson, writer (1850–1894)

What has held you back from reaching your fitness goals in the past? I mean the *real* obstacles? Identifying those stumbling blocks will move you a long way toward resolving them. In fitness, the biggest gains can be made when you turn your mental and physical weaknesses into your strengths. But facing our weaknesses is rarely fun. Now is the time.

One Olympic runner with whom I've trained is relentless in attacking her weaknesses, those things that hold her back from her highest athletic potential. In fact, she rarely works on her strengths. Each week she spends a few moments writing down what holds her back from better fitness, and then she outlines ways to resolve those things immediately. That is why Uta Pippig is one of the most physically, mentally, and psychologically feared athletes in the sport of running.

ACTION ITEM

Write down your biggest physical or mental weaknesses as they relate to your fitness: "knee injury," "no time," "lack of a written program." Then brainstorm a few ideas on how you can address those weaknesses: "Schedule a Friday meeting with Dr. Kelly," "Cut out one hour of television viewing per day," "Create a new written fitness program *right now* and stick it on the fridge." Act on those ideas this week.

4. Write Your Plan and Post It Up

From a good beginning, all else flows.
—DAN MILLMAN, WORLD-CLASS ATHLETE AND AUTHOR

Now that you know why you desire to exercise, it's time to explore how, when, and where. A personalized fitness plan designed by an expert—and you can become that expert—is a road map: it cannot ensure good weather, but it will get you to your destination.

Most people approach their fitness haphazardly. In fact, I know elite-level triathletes who have only a vague idea what exercise they should do each day. They simply throw together a mishmash of workouts and hope for the best. I am a huge fan of spontaneous workouts (see tip #19), but you will get far better results much faster by writing down your plan. Champion athletes build their confidence and successes from adhering to a master success plan. You can, too.

~~~~~~

ACTION ITEM

It's time to create, or rework, your fitness plan. You can build a world-class fitness program in seven simple steps. Pull out a blank sheet of paper and let's get to work!

1. Determine how many hours per week you will dedicate to your new fitness program. Be realistic. It should be no fewer than three. (If you feel that's too much, read tip #85.)

2. Choose two to three rest days. This is vital. No matter what your level or goals, you need at least two days of rest per week. Trust me on this one.

3. Eighty percent of your time should be dedicated to continuous aerobic exercise (cycling, swimming, running, and so on) and 20 percent allocated to strength training. See appendix A for an example of a perfect training week.

4. Two of your aerobic sessions each week are your *key workouts:* one long workout (sixty minutes or more) and one more intense workout. You must be rested for, and recover from, these sessions to boost your fitness.

5. Keep your key workouts as far apart as possible.

6. Post your new program in a highly visible place: mine sits on my refrigerator. The secret of sticking to a new program is being able to see it every day. But that's not enough: you must also write your workouts into your daily planners, so that nobody can take that time from you.

7. Stick to your program, but stay open to modifying it. Your body and mind are dynamic. Therefore the best fitness program is dynamic—changing constantly but subtly, to match how you are feeling each day.

A note to serious athletes: I strongly suggest you consult someone who deeply understands your sport to map out your program. I don't believe most personal trainers at the local gym will cut it. If you were going to ascend Mount Everest, would you hire someone who *studies* the mountain for a living or a team of Sherpas who *climb* that sucker for a living? You need someone who has really "been there, done that." An accomplished athlete in your chosen sport will show you the surest path to your summit while helping you avoid the pitfalls along the way.

5. Redefine "Exercise"

The real voyage of discovery consists not in seeking new landscapes, but in seeing with new eyes.

—MARCEL PROUST, WRITER (1871–1922)

The Tendai "marathon monks" of Japan run one full marathon (26.2 miles) every day for one hundred days as their path to spiritual enlightenment. This is an awe-inspiring physical feat even to professional runners. But the Tendai don't just cover a lot of miles; they see running as much more—each step is another opportunity to learn more about themselves, to go deeper inside. It is their way to complete self-awareness.

In America, most of us don't view exercise that way. Fitness, as part of the national dialogue, has been sadly demoted. We talk about burning calories and chatter about looking thin and managing our weight. We step on the treadmill, hit the green button, turn off our minds, and begin counting.

That is one reason why our exercise doesn't inspire us with the passion it should. When we focus on the superficial benefits of exercise (weight loss, quicker running times), there is an immediate disconnect between body and mind. That makes sticking to a long-term fitness program far more difficult. For the Tendai monks, and for all successful endurance athletes, the calories burned aren't the focus; they are a natural consequence of the passion-driven activity.

The passion and performance approach shifts your perspective. Begin to see each workout session for what it *can* be: a unique opportunity for personal growth, a celebration of life, a walk into the world, part of the total journey. Go out there with a different set of eyes and really open yourself up to the mental and spiritual aspects of exercise. It will be much more valuable to you.

~~~~~~

ACTION ITEM

Step off the treadmill and onto the trails. Even if it means driving an extra twenty minutes, the physical, mental, and spiritual benefits you will experience from exercising in nature is well worth the drive. Get your heart pumping and your endorphins flowing out there. Feel your emotions run deep. Run like the Tendai, and after just a short time your passion will grow and your performance will soar.

6. Do What You Love

~~~~~~

The aim of life is to live, and to live means to be aware, joyously, drunkenly, serenely, divinely aware.

—HENRY MILLER, AUTHOR AND ARTIST (1891–1980)

Your exercise should relate, in some small way, to Henry Miller's philosophy of life. If it doesn't, you're missing out on the magnificent potential exercise has to fill your life with long-lasting passion. Do what you love, and your success in fitness, and in life, is assured. Period. If you take one tip from this book, take this one.

Motivational speaker Tony Robbins often talks about the fundamental driving principle for all human behavior: the pain-pleasure dynamic. According to this theory, every decision is made either to enhance pleasure or to avoid pain. And of the two, the latter is the more powerful force. That may be one reason we struggle with our fitness programs: we simply associate more pain than pleasure with our exercise. To reach new heights of performance and passion, you must begin to associate more exercise with *pleasure*.

Passion is the number one reason why the world's best performers achieve success. *USA Today* reported a study by a Dutch psychologist who tried to figure out what separated chess *grand masters* from mere chess masters. He found no differences in IQ, memory, or spatial reasoning. The only difference? Grand masters had more passion for chess. This is true for every champion athlete I've met, and it applies to your fitness as well.

Three years ago my dad was eighty pounds overweight. The fact that I've *lived* fitness twenty-four hours a day for seven years didn't matter to my dad. He still thinks of me as Bart Simpson. One day we were talking about sports we liked as kids. He mentioned racquetball. I knew that was my chance to change my father's attitude toward fitness. Right then and there, I drove to the sporting goods store and bought the necessary equipment, and we played six fierce games of racquetball at the local YMCA. Today Dad is sixty pounds lighter, and he plays racquetball for three hours a day. He cannot get enough. He goes to bed thinking about it, and he storms out the door in the morning to demolish his buddies on the court. Now *that's* passion for exercise! If you can capture similar feelings about your exercise, you will not fail to reach even your boldest goals.

That is why the absolute bottom line to staying consistent in your fitness program is doing what you love: your exercise should be *passion driven* rather than *guilt induced*. Don't jeopardize your love of exercise for short-term gains. You're not going to feel passionate every time you work out, but you should feel motivated most of the time. If more than five workouts go by without a positive feeling about your exercise, something needs to change.

~~~~~~

ACTION ITEM

There are more sports accessible to you than ever before. Write down five sports you want to try and another five sports you've always loved. They could be rock climbing, group mountain biking, kickboxing. Have you ever tried kickboxing? This could be your favorite sport, but you won't know unless you try! The cardiovascular benefits gained from most aerobic activities are similar, so choose based on passion for the activity rather than on what you think you must do. The point of exercise is to become a fuller, richer human being. Do what you love.

7. Build a Success Journal

~~~~~~

Far better it is to dare mighty things, to win glorious triumphs, even checkered by failure, than to take rank with those poor spirits who neither enjoy much nor suffer much, because they live in the gray twilight that knows not victory nor defeat.

—THEODORE ROOSEVELT, TWENTY-SIXTH PRESIDENT OF THE UNITED STATES (1858–1919)

Making tangible progress in a physical activity that we enjoy motivates and inspires us with confidence. When you can physically see yourself lose weight, run faster, or play longer, your passion for your sport grows. Then you get greedy for more progress. That is the positive cycle top athletes harness in their training programs, and it is the same one you should strive for in your fitness program. You can do this simply by measuring your progress.

Most top athletes use "success journals" to track their fitness gains. By recording workouts over time, they can identify what works and what doesn't in their training and nutrition programs. For example, upon reviewing my success journal, I found that eating peanut-butter sandwiches before workouts produced better, more consistent results. (More on peanut butter and what to eat before and after exercise in tip #57.)

Most important, top athletes use their success journals to boost their confidence when doubts creep in. Some athletes have even been known to pack their journals on trips to big competitions. In the days leading up to the event, they review their best workouts, which instantly dissolves their fear and doubt. It's easy to forget the incredible things you achieve in life, yet it's equally easy to conjure up feelings of confidence just by reviewing what you've done.

Success journals should contain both the physical and the mental successes of your exercise. One entry in my journal read "16-mile run. Incredibly hot. Horseflies were attacking me! First 7 miles great. Forty minutes into the run: dying! Decided to make it a mental toughness session. Amazed I didn't have to stop for the last 5 miles. Anything, absolutely anything, is possible in my life. What's tougher than that run?"

You may feel that recording your exercise is yet another "daily task" added to your already busy life. Don't give in to that feeling. The success journal requires only a few minutes every week, and I've found that it saves me time in the long run by bringing clarity to my fitness program. By reviewing my journal, I learn ways to simplify and streamline my exercise. Plus the confidence I get from having all of my fitness successes in one place is beyond measure. Your success journal will teach you more about your fitness, performance, and passion than any other book you can buy, because it is a book written by you, for you. What could be more valuable and empowering than that?

~~~~~~

ACTION ITEM

Buy a blank notebook, and for the next month record your good training sessions and memorable experiences. Chronicle your successes briefly, but with rich, vivid feeling. You don't need to record every workout, just the ones of particular value and meaning to you. Be sure to write immediately upon completing your workouts, while they are fresh in your mind.

The journal entries will reward you now . . . and later on in life. Periodically glance through your journal, and it will show you why you are a champion in your own right. Sometimes we forget. But it's always in us.

8. Find Peace in the Simplicity of Your Dedication

Success seems to be largely a matter of hanging on after others have let go.
—WILLIAM FEATHER, AUTHOR, *AS WE WERE SAYING* (1921),
AND PUBLISHER (1889–1981)

Now that you are armed with a new program, fresh motivations, and a powerful outlook on your fitness, the question is *How can you stick to that program day in and day out?* The strategies in this book will provide specific ways to ensure that you stay on course, but developing a powerful intrinsic dedication starts with *appreciating the process.*

Some people struggle with the notion of dedicating themselves to a new fitness program. It's seen as another "job." That's one way to see it. The other, better way is that single-mindedly pursuing a new fitness goal can be one of the most rewarding things you will ever do. The famous philosopher Thich Nhat

Hahn said: "When you master one thing, you master everything." After seven years as a professional triathlete, I believe that. Some people ask me what I could possibly get from working out seven hours a day, every day. My answer is always the same: The satisfaction and inner peace I get from pouring my heart into one thing is extraordinary. You can find the same satisfaction and inner peace simply by deepening your dedication to your body.

ACTION ITEM

Committing yourself to building a stronger, healthier body is one of the most virtuous things you can do. Building your body is building a better life for you and the people around you. As you embark on your new fitness program, embrace the *process* and find peace in the simplicity of your wonderful new dedication.

9. Make Illness Prevention the Priority

~~~~~~

One thing that can drain the passion and performance from your life is getting sick. The average American becomes ill twice a year. The following strategies will help you turbocharge your immunity, so that you get sick less—or even not at all! Impossible? Despite training my body into near oblivion on a daily basis, I haven't been sick in five years. There are several reasons why. These techniques are among the most effective:

➤ **Body Awareness.** First, I have learned to tune in so deeply to the signals my body sends that I avoid injury or illness well before it hits. You've heard the quote "When in doubt, cut it out." Apply that to your fitness program. You want to challenge yourself, but you want to avoid pushing past that line. Listen to your body, and it will begin to tell you where that line is. One of the best ways to determine oncoming illness is to check your morning heart rates: an increase of more than ten beats per minute means something is wrong. Another way to predict oncoming illness is to monitor the trends of your benchmark workouts (tip #56).

➤ **Immune Boosters.** At the very first hint of cold or flulike symptoms, you should bombard your body with immune-boosting foods and herbal remedies like garlic, echinacea, vegetable juice, and vitamin C (up to three grams per day). You should also drink as much water as you possibly can. You may want to explore more esoteric methods to boost immunity: hot-cold hydrotherapy, meditation, even "laughter therapy." Laughter produces healthy chemicals in the body and reduces the buildup of the stress chemical cortisol.

➤ **Aerobic Exercise.** This is the most powerful immune booster. Aerobic exercise builds health, strengthens immunity, and just plain makes you feel better. Conversely, extended periods of *anaerobic* exercise wreak havoc on your immune system. The only accurate way to ensure that you are exercising aerobically is to use a heart rate monitor (tip #23).

Make illness prevention a real priority in your life by paying close attention to your body and heeding the warning signals. In the long run, you will be a healthier, fitter, and more passionate human being.

10. Create a Healthy Home

~~~~~~

We spend the majority of our lives at home. It should be a sanctuary of physical, mental, and spiritual replenishment. Top athletes have exceptionally high levels of health and energy. To achieve this, they begin by creating the healthiest possible living spaces they can. Here are a few suggestions I learned from visiting homes of some of the world's best athletes:

➤ Store strong chemicals and cleaning supplies outside of your living space. Our bodies are not equipped to neutralize these chemicals. Toxic chemicals seep into the air we breathe, and this can compromise our health over time.

➤ Don't keep the heat blaring without proper circulation. A hot, stuffy home will make you tired and sick more often since bacteria can more easily "colonize" in such an environment. Keep the windows open, with fresh air flowing through.

➤ Thoroughly declutter your home. This will bring physical and mental clarity to your life. Your lungs will thank you, too.

➤ Buy an ionizer/air filter for your bedroom. Since your body and mind recover most during sleep, it is vital to breathe the freshest possible air during the night.

➤ Play relaxing background music all the time. This can make your home environment much more rejuvenating.

➤ Feng shui deals with how to live in harmony with nature, and its principles can positively influence the way your home looks and feels. Hire an expert or learn how to apply these principles of design yourself.

➤ Oxygenate your home with lots of plants. The best, most resilient "oxygen producers" for the money are spider plants and Boston ferns.

Your work space also deeply influences your overall quality of life. Take a hard, objective look at your work space and decide how you can improve it. Small changes there can lead to significant quality-of-life improvements.

What about spending a little more on a comfortable chair for your back? Hiring an "ergonomic expert"? Finding a place outside where you can take frequent fresh-air breaks? Your employer knows how valuable your health, fitness, and happiness are to the bottom line, so don't be afraid to be bold when making positive changes to your work space.

11. Watch What You Feed Your Mind

The most mentally sound athletes I know are extremely selective about what they read and watch in the news, for good reason. During training and competition, our minds must be perfectly clear of distracting thoughts, and some of the images in today's media are so graphic that we cannot allow that into our minds.

Filtering everything you read and watch may be a little extreme for most people, but it does underlie an important concept: We become a literal "repository" of everything we see, hear, and do. Today more than ever, we're bombarded with negative images and stories on such a repeated basis, who knows what seeps into our subconscious? If you want to perform at a higher level and amplify your passion for life, you should seriously look at the effects the mass media has on your mental fitness.

Your mind is the most priceless thing you will ever own. Broadly speaking, does the daily television and print news really enrich your overall long-term health, happiness, and passion for life? Take some time to decide if mass media is something you want to "soak up" on a daily basis. It's important to stay abreast of the human condition, but you can make a difference in the world without letting the media negatively and constantly influence your daily frame of mind.

12. Commit to Getting Pain Free Once and for All

How on earth can you live with passion and perform as a human being if you're in pain? Pain is insidious because we are so skilled at adapting to and working around it. Imperceptibly, over time, we simply learn to live with pain, which when you think objectively about it seems a little crazy, doesn't it? It's time to find permanent solutions to your pain. And you are a lot closer to resolving pain issues than you might think.

Clearly the most desirable step is to avoid injury altogether. Most injuries can be prevented simply by listening to your body, which will send warning signals well in advance of injury. Preventative therapies like chiropractic, deep-tissue massage, yoga, and acupuncture are among the best ways to "tune in to" your body and create a more resilient physique.

If you get injured, the most valuable thing you can do is get an accurate diagnosis immediately, so that you do not inadvertently make the injury worse—such as applying heat when you should apply ice. I cannot overstress the importance of seeking the advice of someone who deeply understands the nature of your pain or injury, as opposed to someone who simply claims to understand. Early in my career I injured my lower back, and it almost drove me out of the sport. I stretched, strengthened, and iced that injury constantly. I saw countless doctors and physical therapists around the world. None of them helped. Then I heeded the advice of a top pro athlete and called Dr. Walter Lightner, a specialist based in Corte Madera, California. In twenty minutes Dr. Lightner indicated that I had a "chronic muscle tear." The treatment: No stretching and no heat. That would just retear and inflame the injury. I needed deep-tissue bodywork to realign the muscle fibers, at which point I could stretch again. Had I met Walter Lightner four years earlier, I would've saved hundreds of hours, tens of thousands of dollars, and untold heartache. Please, find real experts to address your pain and injury issues.

A final note: Try to rely less on drugs you take for pain. Drugs simply mask your problem, and they don't move you closer to a final resolution of your injury. Instead of treating a problem symptomatically with drugs, dig deep to find out what's causing your problem.

ACTION ITEM

Do a thorough rundown of your body, head to toe. What has been hurting you for more than a month? Next consult an expert, a proven expert (tip #68), and map out a strategy to resolve your pain. I assure you that when you achieve a fully pain-free body, your passion and performance will absolutely sky-rocket.

13. Move Your Body to Move Your Mind

You've heard the saying "Motion creates emotion." This is absolutely true. The best way to sharpen your mind is to shift your body, and the world's best athletes prove it.

Before major international competitions, I would always see the top pros prancing around like peacocks. I couldn't figure this out, because I was always so nervous that the entire lower half of my body would grow numb! Not the best way to gear up for a triathlon event. To my delight, I later discovered most of the pros were just as nervous as I was, but by "acting as if" they were confident, they grew to believe they were. This is one of the most common strategies champion athletes use to achieve the mental frame of mind needed for world-class performances. It's very easy to learn.

Right now, sit or stand up straight, take in a deep, full breath through your nose, and put a smile on your face. Come on, nobody is watching. And if they are, maybe your positive energy will rub off on them. Now, when you are in this position, how do you feel? Your mood and energy level should improve noticeably. It's difficult to remain depressed, tired, or frustrated for too long while your body is in an energetic position. Practice this often. Move your body to move your mind.

14. Your Warm-up Determines Your Workout

Warm-ups often get short shrift, but your warm-up may be the most important part of your workout, setting the tone for your entire exercise session.

Most people feel that they simply don't have time to warm up: "I've only got thirty minutes. Better get out there and hammer away." You will never in a million years see a professional athlete do this—the warm-up is far too important to performance and injury prevention. It's not that you don't have the time to warm up, you don't have the time *not to warm up*.

"The World's Fittest Man," Mark Allen, walks for four blocks before every run. If he gives that much reverence to warming up, you can, too. Proper warm-ups prevent injury, burn more fat during exercise, increase athletic performance, and make exercise feel noticeably easier.

Your warm-up need not be complex. For the first ten minutes of your workout, go nice and easy and breathe deeply and slowly. If you begin to run out of breath during the warm-up, you're going way too hard. Some top athletes perform what they call a "stop and go" warm-up, which I've found to be quite effective at getting the body ready for a great workout. Here's how it works: Begin your exercise for a few minutes very easily and then stop for ten to twenty seconds. Start up for another three minutes, then take another thirty-second rest. Continue that process through the ten-minute warm-up. This gradual "ramping up" of your aerobic system allows your body to pump the blood more efficiently, which oxygenates your muscles better than if you were to dive right into the workout. You know you're probably warmed up when you break a sweat.

ACTION ITEM

The next time you exercise, give a little more attention to your warm-up. Take the time to ease into your workout. If you have only thirty minutes to exercise, it's better for your body to warm up for ten minutes, run steadily for fifteen, and cool down for five.

15. Be Bad

I'd rather laugh with the sinners than cry with the saints.
—BILLY JOEL, SINGER/SONGWRITER

This one stopped you dead in your tracks, didn't it. That's because we all like to be bad—once in a while, at least.

If the eighties were about overindulgence, the nineties were about deprivation. These days you're not allowed to eat anything: sugar, fats, carbohydrates, meat—even water will kill you. How can you live with more passion and perform if you are in a perpetual state of paranoia and deprivation?

Many people lose the motivation to stick to higher nutrition or fitness programs because they just can't be "good" indefinitely. Nobody can. The secret to lifelong fitness success is to be bad on an infrequent but regular basis. It's the only way the body and mind can cope with the demands of a higher-quality fitness program.

Take Australia's Greg Welch, clearly one of the best triathletes who ever lived. He has won every world championship there is. He also drove his competition crazy. Welch is one of the most affable, down-to-earth athletes you will ever meet. Before major international competitions, he would relax with a few beers and a lot of laughs. While he enjoyed himself the night before the event, I would remain holed up in my hotel room, taking hot baths, elevating my legs, and practicing my victory speech. On race day, Welch would invariably, unequivocally, kick my butt. I couldn't crack that Aussie nut. Finally I decided to learn from him.

When Welch is bad, he's really bad. He enjoys his beers and his chocolate cake. But when he's good, he's absolutely focused and down to business. It's as if Welch's downtime powers his uptime. Does that make sense? Those times of relaxation provide the mental and physical break he needs to get back to training with more passion and resolve the next day. And Welch never feels guilty about missing a workout; he uses it as positive fuel.

As you begin to exercise smarter, it's important to reward yourself on a regular basis. You may want to eat well six days out of the week and on that seventh day let all the rules go. Order a pizza or have a few scoops of Ben & Jerry's ice cream. This doesn't give you license to go ballistic and eat five pizzas. It's just that in the long run balanced living is healthier than an unblemished eating record. Be bad once in a while in your fitness program—you will begin to associate more pleasure than pain with your exercise, and that leads to greater long-term success.

16. What Matters Is Not the Number of Hours You Put In, but What You Put into Those Hours

The "more is better" work ethic does not apply to your fitness program. This is one of the most common misconceptions about exercise that can be very destructive to your passion and performance.

Exercising too often or too strenuously is a sure path to burnout. You may achieve excellent short-term results, but you jeopardize your future fitness. You will perform better and have more passion for your exercise if you focus *more* on *fewer* workouts. What do I mean?

From now on, aim for quality over quantity. Think *smarter*, not *harder*. Whatever your fitness level or goals, all you generally need is four days of exercise per week. That's it. Even at the peak of my training for the Ironman Triathlon, I was training only five days a week. The other two days were vital for mental and physical convalescence.

However, I learned the "less is more" lesson the hard way. After achieving success early in my career, I got greedy and increased my training time to over forty-five hours per week. If twenty-five hours a week earned me a number six world ranking, surely forty-five would be enough to win a world championship. Needless to say, this led to my demise. Over the next two years, I didn't have a single decent performance. Having put in a Herculean amount of work, I found that a tough statistic to take. But there was something far more damaging to my performance: I lost the love for my sport. I had literally "trained" the passion out of myself.

Most people don't train forty-five hours per week, but the lesson applies just the same. As you begin to achieve new fitness results, your passion will grow—and that's good. You may begin to feel a tendency to do more. Don't. View your fitness as a long-term journey up a mountain path. To continue moving up, you must ration your time and energy. Remember, you will be exercising for decades to come. This long-term vision will help ensure that you don't overdo it and train yourself into the ground.

17. Experience the Perfect Workout

We all want to get the maximum benefit from the time we spend exercising. To get the most from every workout, here are a few simple things you should do before, during, and after each session that will boost its effects:

1. Have a workout goal. Knowing your physical or mental goal for each workout before you begin sets in motion the desired results almost immediately.

2. Eat the right foods beforehand. As we explain in greater detail in tip #57, what you eat before your exercise has a large impact on how well your body and mind will perform during the session. Eat predominantly quality fat and proteins before and carbos and sugars after. A peanut-butter sandwich an hour before a workout is perfect, because it will sustain you physically and mentally. In addition, to maintain steady blood sugar levels during exercise, it's best not to eat within thirty minutes before workouts.

3. Warm up longer. Be sure to give at least ten minutes to easing into your workout. This prevents injury, increases performance, and literally makes the workout feel easier (see tip #14).

4. Focus on your breathing and technique. This is the best way to keep your focus sharp and your performance up. The world's best athletes concentrate almost exclusively on these two elements during training and racing, and for good reason. The common mantra of many top athletes during competition is "Breathe, flow, technique." Keep your breathing deep and rhythmical and maintain good technique. The quality of your workouts will soar.

5. Monitor your intensity. Some people have little idea how hard to go during a workout. The secret is to stick to four general levels of exercise (see tip #24), and the only way to accurately gauge your exercise intensity is to use a heart rate monitor (see tip #23).

6. Stay hydrated and well fueled. Dehydration is insidious. Just a 2 percent drop in your body's water levels can lead to a 10 percent decline in performance. Drink one standard water bottle and consume 40–60 grams of carbohydrate per hour during exercise. You'll work out better and recover more quickly.

7. Warm down for five minutes. A cool-down will "flush" your muscles of the waste products that build up in your body during exercise. This will help you recover and make your next session feel easier.

8. Eat well immediately afterward to maximize recovery. Your body is most receptive to nutrients directly after a workout. Eat something substantial after tough exercise.

18. Quiet Your Mind During Workouts

A mind too active is no mind at all.
—THEODORE ROETHKE, POET (1908–1963), *STRAW FOR THE FIRE: FROM THE NOTEBOOKS OF THEODORE ROETHKE*, 1943–1963

When we quiet the mind, the symphony begins.
—ANONYMOUS

A quiet mind translates into inner peace. Inner peace opens us up to more passion and greater performance. When we calm our minds, our bodies follow—and that is when we physically operate at our best. Learning this technique will do wonders for your mental and spiritual fitness.

Quieting the mind for long periods of time is tough, in part because modern society has subverted our ability to calm the inner chatter. Our minds are active all day, like a car running at 6,000 rpm for sixteen hours a day. But I have found a place where my mind relaxes every time, and it's where I perform best: nature. For me, running, hiking, or biking in the forest is cathartic. Invariably, by the end of these sessions, life's "irreconcilable problems" are brought into focus. There is something about exercising in the absence of society that brings out our most uninhibited, creative thoughts, and our deepest peace of mind, our most passionate self.

As you learn to quiet your mind during easy exercise, apply that skill to more intense workouts. This can be enormously effective at increasing your athletic performance. I didn't reach my true potential as an athlete until I learned to race with complete mindlessness. At one race in Japan, something extraordinary happened to me. I was halfway through the one-hundred-kilometer bike portion of the triathlon, in third place. I was thinking of every reason why I was not winning: inconsistent training habits, dehydration, even the ice cream I'd had the night before. It must have shown on my face, because coming into a slow uphill turn, I locked eyes with an old woman who almost whispered to me as I rode by: "Let your mind go, you're thinking too much." It gave me the chills. It was so powerful, my mind just shut off right on the spot. From that point on, I raced without thought, and before I knew it, I was breaking the finishing tape in the first major victory of my professional career.

Try this simple exercise. Throw an object into the air and catch it. Do you remember how you felt while the object was in the air? Probably not, because between the throw and the catch, you experienced satori—the complete mindless focus that champion athletes have during world-record performances. Their body is the hurricane and their mind is the eye. That is the level of mindlessness you should strive for during your exercise.

~~~~~~

ACTION ITEM

The next time you work out, seek out the most beautiful setting you can find and walk, run, or cycle there, whatever gets your heart pumping—literally and figuratively. After about five minutes wipe all of the thoughts from your mind and move toward that state of satori. If there is something bothering you, don't fight it, just move it aside and continue exercising. This is a high-level skill that will lead to more enjoyable, more effective, workouts.

19. Don't Work Out, Play Out

Surrender doesn't obstruct our power; it enhances it.
—MARIANNE WILLIAMSON, AUTHOR, *A RETURN TO LOVE* (1996)

We do not stop playing because we grow old; we grow old because we stop playing.
—ANONYMOUS

When did we stop playing and start "working out"? I suspect it happened some time in our late teens or early twenties. Exercise became another form of work. That's too bad, because physical activity is not meant to be work. You *work* enough! In fact, from now on "working out" might usefully be referred to as "playing out." It's time to get out there and play again.

When we were children, physical activity was all about play: kickball, tag, boogie-boarding, whatever. We would spend hours, without thought, *playing* our favorite sport. We did it for one reason: It was fun.

That pure passion for physical activity is one reason we were so energetic as children, why we slept so soundly, why we were always so full of excitement. We were simply using our bodies all the time—which is central to living a passion-filled life. If you can recapture that present-moment passion, that childlike innocence about physical activity, you will reach heights of passion and performance you never dreamed possible.

You may think you've lost the ability to play, but you're wrong. I can prove it. Think about the last time you played your favorite sport. You probably felt more like a child then than you do in your daily life. You were fully immersed in the activity, and for moments there, you relinquished your self-consciousness. *That's* where you want to strive to be during workouts. Remember, physical activity is physical activity—you derive the same aerobic benefit from something fun like basketball that you do from something that may bore you, such as the StairMaster.

Serious athletes take note. For me, when triathlon became solely a business, I hated it and I performed far worse. *My passion drained out, and my performance tanked!* It took me three years to learn one of the most important lessons: When you loosen up, your mind and body will produce far more impressive results.

~~~~~~

ACTION ITEM

During your next few workouts, try to recapture the feelings you had as a child—if only for fleeting moments. Be passionate out there and spontaneous. You can still be serious about your sport, just don't let anyone or anything pierce your idyllic reverie during your "play-outs!" The only rule is that you must let go of all rules and expectations. "Playing" takes practice, but it will reward you on many levels. It may even make you feel like a child again.

20. Modify Your Goals and Clarify Your Motivations

To improve is to change. To be perfect is to change often.

—WINSTON CHURCHILL, BRITISH PRIME MINISTER AND STATESMAN (1874–1965)

Specific goals are the physical stepping-stones to your dreams, but when you lose steam, you must be willing to pull back and reassess what you are doing and why. Your body and mind are wonderfully dynamic, and regimented fitness programs do not always produce the best possible results.

Your goals and your motivations may change every month. That's okay. It doesn't mean you're giving up; you're just listening to your body and mind. For example, you may discover that you've had enough of swimming and you want to power-hike for the next month. Great. As long as your fitness goals remain equally passionate and ambitious, go ahead and change directions.

Remember, introducing different sports or exercises leads to mental growth and physical balance.

The best way to determine when you need to modify your fitness goals and reclarify your motivations is to ask this question: *How long has it been since I've been really excited to work out?* If you have not been genuinely excited to reach your fitness goals (tip #1) and are not doing what you love (tip #6) *for more than four workouts,* it's time for a change.

Once you decide you need a change, whip out a blank sheet of paper and reformulate your goals just as you did in tip #1. Then, if necessary, choose another sport or exercise to do for the next couple of months. I've found that kickboxing usually provides me with a good shot of passion and a needed break from my primary sport of triathlon.

21. Be Present

Life becomes more precious when there's less of it to waste.

—BONNIE RAITT, SINGER/SONGWRITER

It cannot be bought; it cannot be "earned"; it cannot be created by any means; and it cannot be retrieved once it is gone. Therefore *time* is our most precious commodity, and we must protect it as if our lives depend on it.

I try to live my life as if I were a ninety-year-old temporarily sent back into the body of a twenty-nine-year-old. This forces me to live fully in every moment. By training tens of thousands of hours, I've mastered the art of "slowing time" during exercise, which is a skill you can learn as well. Present-moment awareness during exercise can "give" you more time. By slowing down and paying attention to each moment, you can transform a simple one-hour workout into a richly rewarding, timeless experience. Learning this important skill releases a treasure trove of new adventures and passion, and it is probably the most valuable skill you can take from physical activity into daily life. Many famous philosophers believe that present-moment awareness is fundamental to a happy, successful life.

~~~~~~

ACTION ITEM

Nowhere can one practice present-moment awareness better than during solitary exercise somewhere in nature. Perform your next workout outside, and quiet your mind. Open your senses wide: hear the birds, feel your heartbeat, smell the fragrances around you, picture your lungs taking in the air and distributing it to your working muscles. When you are fully present in the moment, your passion will come alive, time will fall away, and you will open yourself up to an exciting level of performance. This is what champion athletes experience during competition: senses fully alive, mind completely quiet. (See tip #18 about quieting the mind.)

Once you master this skill during exercise, apply it to your life. Be present in whatever you do: it will lead to better physical performance and a greater appreciation of what were once ordinary moments in your life.

22. Stop Counting Calories

The original name for this tip was "For the Love of God, Stop Counting Calories and Limiting Calorie Intake. Just Eat When You Feel Real Hunger." The reason is that this technique will allow you to make the right food decisions at the right times. Not only will this liberate your mind and body from calorie-counting craziness, you will begin to trust yourself on issues beyond food. That self-empowerment is what this book is all about.

There are countless people out there telling you how and what to eat, and all of them forget one incontrovertible truth: *You* are the foremost authority on your body. Stored in your genetic code are all the answers you need to make the best possible food choices.

From now on, food cannot be measured in calories. It must be measured in level of nourishment. Begin to tune in to your inner hunger signals and trust yourself on food choices. When you feel hungry, think about what is best to eat at that time and in what amounts. Then eat slowly and stop when you feel satisfied. We're so accustomed to believing that "diet changes" need to be revolutionary in order to make a difference in our lives that the strategy presented here may appear far too simplistic. However, it is the healthiest and most permanent way to control your eating, bar none. This is a tough skill to develop, but you can do it with practice. Learning to rely on your body's signals about food will save you untold amounts of time, money, and frustration. Most important, it will empower *you* more than a nutrition expert ever can.

23. Buy a Heart Rate Monitor

This may be the most important fitness tip in the book. A heart monitor will give anyone at any fitness level the most possible benefit from the time spent exercising. Period. Exercising without one is exercising blindly. Six-time Ironman champion Dave Scott, arguably one of the fittest people in the world, says of heart monitors: "Every question I ever had about exercise or training was answered when I bought, and began using, a heart rate monitor." I agree.

Quick physiology lesson: Heart rate is the most accurate measure of how hard your body is working during exercise and at rest. That is why a heart rate monitor is so integral to achieving health, fitness, and athletic results. As you become fitter, your heart becomes stronger—it can pump more blood with each beat, allowing you to do the same work at the lower effort levels. This is the essence of aerobic fitness.

A heart rate monitor also serves as a compliance tool, a literal personal coach that "monitors" you during workouts. Most monitors have high and low "alarms" that will sound if you are exercising too hard or not hard enough.

A heart monitor will also help you predict oncoming illness and overtraining. By learning how your heart performs in certain situations (say, at rest, at twenty miles per hour on the bike, or at a seven-minute-per-mile pace while running), you can identify when your heart is beating abnormally high—and that means it's time for a rest. This is probably a heart monitor's biggest value, since it can keep you healthy and strong all year long. Using a heart monitor to predict oncoming illness is one strategy top athletes use to stay healthy despite training thousands of hours per year.

The basis of heart rate exercise is your "anaerobic threshold" (AT). For most people this represents, in heartbeats per minute, the point at which your body shifts from using fat as fuel to using sugar. To determine your AT, first subtract your age from 180. This is the starting point. Now, during your next workout, push just to the point at which you run out of breath. Record that number on your heart rate monitor. This "ventilory threshold" usually coincides with your anaerobic threshold, so take the average of these two numbers. That is your *true AT*, and it is the only number you need to know for exercise. It will change over time and across sports, so check your AT every couple of weeks. Now that you know your true AT, to get the most from your exercise, simply work out in four different "zones," each of which produces different physiological results. That's what the next strategy will cover.

~~~~~~

ACTION ITEM

Do some research and decide if this technology is for you. If it is, log on to www.BodyFire.com—they sell the best heart rate monitors at the lowest prices.

24. Exercise in Four Zones

~~~~~~

One of the most confusing parts of exercise is knowing how hard to go to achieve your desired result. The simplest answer to this is, just view your exercise intensity in terms of four zones.

To determine your personal target zones, use your true anaerobic threshold, calculated in the previous tip. Let's use a forty-year-old woman with an AT of 140 beats per minute as the example in determining the four levels of exercise:

Level I—Recovery: The purpose of level I exercise is to just get out there, have some fun, and build general aerobic fitness without fatigue. Your effort level should be "easy." Heart rates should not exceed 120 beats per minute.

Level II—Aerobic/"Fat Burning": This is where you should spend the vast majority of your exercise time. Level II exercise builds aerobic fitness, strengthens immunity, and burns body fat as the primary source of fuel. Heart rates for this level: 110–140 beats per minute.

Level III—Intervals: When your aerobic fitness begins to plateau (tip #56), it's time to dash some intervals into your workouts. These intervals can last anywhere from thirty seconds to eight minutes. Subjective effort level is "comfortably challenging": you should feel like working fairly hard, but you should *not* feel out of control. Heart rates will be in the 140–155 range.

Level IV—Maximal Efforts: These are reserved for people who want high-end fitness, particularly competitive athletes. Efforts should be from five seconds to thirty seconds in duration and should be at just about an all-out effort. These sessions will dramatically improve your maximal-oxygen-carrying capacity and your biomechanical technique.

Generally, each week you should have two level II workouts, one level I workout, and one level III workout. When you feel that you want to reach the next level in your fitness, one level IV workout every two weeks is plenty.

25. Channel Negative Emotions into Positive Action

Master this skill and there is little you cannot do in your life. Just as the feelings of fear, anger, and frustration can render us powerless, they can motivate each of us to world-class performances. Don't believe me? Imagine you're strolling along in the forest. You glance up and realize you've come between a mother bear and her cubs. No matter who you are, how old you are, or how fit you are, I guarantee, you will run five-minute miles in the opposite direction. And that's world-class speed. That is what fear can do, and if you learn to channel negative emotions like fear into positive action, you will perform at a much higher level, in workouts and in life.

Before the start of my biggest athletic events, I would see a few pros getting sick because they were so nervous. Twenty minutes later they were performing with dazzling grace and power. Somewhere along the way, they had transformed their fear into calm, powerful, efficient action. You can learn this skill with a little practice.

~~~~~~

ACTION ITEM

I learned this technique from a Finnish cross-country skier who uses negative emotions as fuel during workouts and competitions: The next time you work out, pick a couple of things that are really bothering you. Assign a color to those negative emotions—say, red. This is your "workout fuel." As you begin to work out, visualize that powerful red jet fuel pouring into your heart, your legs, and your lungs. Let those feelings fuel your passion. Now *focus* that fuel into efficient forward motion: be as calm, strong, and focused as possible. Picture the red fuel burning off as you work out. As you cool-down, picture an "empty tank" and let all of the remaining red fuel just evaporate into the air.

Normally it's best to be positively motivated to exercise, but don't underestimate the value of burning off negative energy in a positive way during exercise.

26. Volunteer Just One Day at a Special Olympics

I've trained and raced with the most finely honed athletes on the planet—people who forge passion into performance and performance into greatness. As dazzling as these athletes are, they can't hold a candle to what unfolds at the Special Olympics.

The athletes who compete here are unique in that they are purely passionate about their sports. Performance is not based on high-dollar contracts or public adulation. This is about clean, unadulterated passion, which is what makes this competition and these athletes so singular in the athletic world.

One story sticks out in my mind as representative of the passion and humanity of the Special Olympics. It was the one-hundred-meter final. Eight well-oiled athletes toed the line, as intent on winning as any Olympic champion. The gun exploded, as did the legs and arms of these athletes. Halfway through the race, one athlete fell to the ground. He was so grief-stricken, he began to cry. The other athletes, hearing their fallen competitor, all stopped, turned around, and made sure he was okay. They *all* stopped. And they did so without reservation and in total concert. Furthermore, they insisted that the race begin again, and this time they all crossed the line. It was one of the greatest displays of sportsmanship I've ever witnessed.

~~~~~~

ACTION ITEM

Log on to www.specialolympics.org and get involved with a Special Olympics in your area. Open up your heart, and these people will teach you all about pure passion and performance.

27. Supercharge Your Workouts

hampion athletes spend years developing new, high-horsepower fitness techniques. There are a few things top athletes do that can bring your workouts to another level. Here are a few suggestions:

➤ Learn active isolated stretching (AIS). This cutting-edge, dynamic stretch routine will increase your joint and muscle flexibility as much as anything you will ever do. It requires only a rope and ten minutes a day. The best book on AIS is *The Whartons' Stretch Book: Featuring the Breakthrough Method of Active-Isolated Stretching* (Times Books, 1996).

➤ Use your heart rate monitor in more advanced ways: watch how long it takes for your heart rate to come down after hard efforts—the best measure of fitness is how quickly you recover. Record your waking heart rates to detect oncoming illness and overtraining. Test out new techniques during workouts to see how they affect the amount of power you can put out at a given heart rate.

➤ Videotape yourself. The best way to improve your technique in your chosen sport is to watch yourself on video. You don't need to be a world-class athlete to benefit from this powerful strategy, because seeing yourself perform helps you develop a better body awareness no matter what your fitness level. Watch the world's best athletes and apply what you see the next time you perform your sport.

➤ Drink one to two cups of strong coffee or, better yet, green tea one hour before workouts; 200–300 mg caffeine will burn more body fat, sharpen your focus, and expand your aerobic capacity.

➤ During workouts, breathe deep into your belly as opposed to "panting" into your upper chest (tip #64). The greatest oxygen exchange takes place in the lower areas of your lungs.

➤ Work out with others. You will put in more time and effort when exercising with another than you are normally willing to give alone. For more on that, read the next tip.

28. Buddy Up

Our moods, habits, and level of performance naturally gravitate to the people with whom we spend the most time. This is particularly true of fitness. If you work out with encouraging people who challenge you physically, mentally, or spiritually in some way, you will get a great deal more from exercise. That is why *whom* you choose as your workout buddies will not only determine your long-term success, it will also determine how much you enjoy the process.

Since we are social creatures, social facilitation powerfully influences the way we work out. In most cases, we will give more to a workout when we do it with others. In addition, we are less willing to skip a workout if others are relying on us. For these two reasons, I rarely miss group workouts.

Begin to cultivate a strong network of workout buddies who care about fitness and exercise with passion. Revel in the competition, the camaraderie, and the thrill of the group dynamic. You may even want to make a deal with your new workout buddies, committing to a quest for higher fitness. Keep a list of their numbers handy. When your motivation is down or your exercise needs a lift, give your buddies a call and get out that door.

29. Loosen Up

If you are doing your best, you will not have to worry about failure.
—ROBERT HILLYER, POET (1895–1961)

Frustration comes from expectation. Think about it. When you're most frustrated, you generally see the way things *should be,* but you are stuck in a place far from that vision. That's why I get so aggravated while sitting in traffic—I know where I should be . . . oh, I can see it. *But I won't get there until these people in front of me move in a forward direction. . . .*

A Japanese sumo wrestler gave me great advice on expectation. First, we genuinely must "accept that we, and life, are imperfect." Then he explained that "clearly knowing your task at hand, letting go of expectation, and doing your best will leave no room for worry or frustration." He stressed that it was about accepting the way things are *without getting ambivalent or relaxing our standards.*

~~~~~~

ACTION ITEM

In fitness, it's important to have clear, ambitious goals (tip #1), but don't get so tied to the end result that you are in a constant state of frustration. Fitness is a process. Ironically, if you just loosen up and focus on the here and now, before you know it, you will arrive at your destination and the journey will have been enjoyed.

30. Learn to Hear and Obey Messages from Your Body

This is one of the most important tips in the book, because it puts you in charge of your body and your life. Developing keen body sensitivity is one of the crucial things you can do to achieve better levels of fitness. It allows you to "coach" yourself as opposed to looking outside for answers. The best athletes in the world rely on their inner coach even more than their real-world coaches.

How do we develop this body awareness? Watch animals in action. They have perfect body awareness. Have you ever seen a cat stretch? If a cat feels tight, it will s-t-r-e-t-c-h until if feels j-u-u-u-s-t right. When a dog is sleepy, he rests his entire body. Animals are completely in touch with how their bodies feel, and they act on those feelings without thought. We have that same instinctual ability to know what's best for our bodies, but our go-go lifestyle often subverts that. Begin to "tune in" to your body on a more regular basis and you'll begin to hear the messages it's sending.

It's not enough simply to *hear* the signals from your body, you must become accustomed to *acting* on them without thought. It's about being more instinctual and less concerned with what others think. I'm an extreme example of this: if my back is sore, I will plop right down and stretch wherever I am. People sometimes stare in amazement, but I cannot imagine their bodies are tension free. If they could let go of their self-consciousness, they would plop down on the floor and join me.

~~~~~~

ACTION ITEM

Begin to clear up the communication channels with yourself by pausing throughout the day and "taking stock" of your body. Questions to ask yourself every hour or so are *Are my muscles relaxed? Am I breathing deeply? How's my energy level: do I need to eat or drink?* Once you open up the dialogue between your mind and your body, learn to take immediate action on the signals your body is sending.

31. Choose Better Exercise Venues

It's a big world, yet many of us, including yours truly, confine our workouts to very limited spaces. The environment in which we exercise determines, in large part, our passion for that activity and how well we perform. Here are a few suggestions on choosing the best possible venues to exercise:

➤ Choose to exercise in a beautiful natural setting whenever given the chance. The mental and spiritual benefits you will reap from connecting with yourself in nature are equivalent to the physical benefits of aerobic exercise. Workouts in nature give you triple the bang for your buck.

➤ Do not exercise near congested traffic. It's better to sit on the couch than to breathe car exhaust for an hour. In addition, the risk of injury increases dramatically when you mix exercise with cars.

➤ Exercise outdoors in the cold or the rain, but not in both. It takes too great a toll on your body. However, easy exercise in light rain can be very exhilarating.

➤ Change your workout venues often. Without knowing it, we grow stale from exercising in the same place over and over again. Every couple of weeks, seek out new places, and new adventures will follow.

32. Music Is a Powerful Motivator

While training overseas, I ran across the two-hundred-meter gold medalist Michael Johnson on the track. More precisely, he ran by me at an embarrassingly fast pace. What struck me about Michael, other than his divine stride and motionless upper body, was the heavy bass of rap music pouring out of his Walkman. Between intervals I asked him about this. Michael Johnson uses powerful music to stir his passion to the boiling point; then he releases his passion in training and competition. You too can use music to motivate you before and during all of your workouts.

The first step is to find music that really moves you. I mean stuff that gives you *chills*. What music makes you want to jump out the door and exercise? If it's the theme to *Rocky*, then go with it. That's the music you need to listen to before and, if appropriate, during workouts. For me, it's the pounding rhythm of the Crystal Method, a band that plays a new style of music called "techno." I reserve this strong, rhythmical music for my most important workouts.

~~~~~~

Create your own workout tapes. Since your body will generally follow the intensity level of the music you are listening to, be sure that the first ten minutes of your tapes consist of easy music. For the main part of your workout, choose steady-state music with a good beat. Some researchers have found that music running at 60–90 cpm (cycles per minute) induces alpha waves in the brain. During your musically enhanced workouts, focus on the music, your technique, and your breathing and watch your passion and performance soar.

33. Practice Doesn't Make Perfect— Perfect Practice Makes Perfect

Most elite-level athletes have equivalent levels of fitness, but the champions separate themselves with superior biomechanical technique. Take Tiger Woods. By most standards he's a fairly average-looking athletic guy. How is it that Tiger outdrives the world's best professional golfers by such a large margin? Many attribute it to his technique—some believe that he simply builds up a little extra torque through a highly flexible prerelease of his hips.

This isn't about trying to become a world-class athlete. It's about performing a skill with more grace and fluidity, which can be exhilarating no matter what your fitness level or goals. Subtle improvements in your technique will prevent injury and increase your performance, particularly in repetitive sports like cycling, swimming, or running. For example, if you learned to increase your stride length just one-half inch, you would take up to twenty minutes off your marathon time.

Refining your technique is a simple and powerful way to boost the performance and enjoyment of your physical activity. Watch the top players in your sport and mimic their movements. Aim to perform your chosen skill perfectly, at least once. When you feel what it's like to execute a skill flawlessly, you will develop a much more controlled body awareness. To accelerate this process, you may want to get some hands-on attention from an expert in your chosen activity.

34. Focus on the Solution More Than the Problem

What is defeat? Nothing but education; nothing but the first step to something better.
—RICHARD SHERIDAN, PLAYWRIGHT (1751–1816)

It is easy to let ourselves get wrapped up in the problem rather than focusing on the solution. I've watched some people obsess with their problem so much, it's almost as if talking about it *soothes them*. I suspect that's because problems are concrete; we can identify them easily, and that provides the illusion of control: "I'm ten pounds overweight" or "I'll never run a six-minute mile." The solution, on the other hand, is multifaceted: it requires honesty, creativity, determination, patience, and focus.

The best athletes don't focus on their problems. In fact, the true champions recognize problems and map out the solutions immediately. Tour de France champion Lance Armstrong is the classic example of this. When he learned that he had cancer, among Lance's first thoughts were "Okay. I will beat this. What do I need to do right now and over the next week, month, and year to eradicate this from my body?" And he did. Lance was completely focused on the solution and absolutely tireless in pursuing it. Had he spent too much time focused on the problem, he might not be alive today.

~~~~~~

ACTION ITEM

When you come up against an obstacle or challenge, in a workout or in daily life, take a deep breath through your nose (tip #64) and turn your attention to the solution. Understand the problem, but spend the majority of your time and energy on the solution.

35. Morning Workouts Are Best

My most rewarding and effective workouts were performed at the first light of day. Even if it means you must wake up at a very early hour, you will find that exercising in the morning can enhance your life just as much as your fitness, because it provides an uninterrupted time of peaceful solitude.

Here's what will happen if you exercise in the mornings:

➤ You will miss workouts less often.
➤ You will burn more body fat. As I've mentioned in this book, blood sugar and insulin levels can determine the quality of your workouts. When you wake up in the morning, your insulin levels are steadier, which translates into more body fat burned during morning workouts.
➤ The solitude and peace your morning sessions provide will create a more balanced, centered frame of mind all day.

➤ Your day will be more productive. Aerobic exercise clears your head and energizes your body. The caveat to this is that you must exercise aerobically (tip #67). If you cross over into the anaerobic zone, you will feel cloudy, tired, and even cranky for the remainder of the day.

~~~~~~

ACTION ITEM

Begin to move some of your workouts to the mornings. This week get up early and get right out that door. Just go. Sometimes that extra hour of peaceful solitude is worth the missed hour of sleep. Some of the best experiences can be had by exercising at first light. It's also nice to know that by eight A.M. you've done more than some people do all week!

36. Develop an Unflappable Self-Esteem

No person who is occupied in doing a very difficult thing, and doing it very well, ever loses his self-respect.

—GEORGE BERNARD SHAW, WRITER (1856–1950)

The most permanent and powerful way I've learned to build a rock-solid self-esteem is to build my body. When you have followed an effective fitness plan, your body will show the effects of that, and you will radiate confidence. But you must commit to your fitness program 100 percent, since the amount you trust yourself is in direct proportion to your ability to keep promises to yourself.

As I trained for triathlons, the one thing that progressively grew in me, regardless of setbacks, performance, or outside opinion, was my self-esteem. In chronicling all of my successes, small and large (tip #7), my self-esteem grew steadily to the point where *I believed I could do anything.* You can parlay your small fitness successes into a durable self-esteem that will serve you in daily life.

~~~~~~

ACTION ITEM

On a week that you have relatively more free time, perform your chosen exercise or sport with great intention. Write out a one-week plan that is realistic but challenging, and stick to it. Just for one week. Record every workout that you do. When you are focused on a goal and pursue that goal, especially in exercise or sport, your self-esteem will strengthen from the inside out—and nobody can take that from you.

37. Juice Up Your Performance

The simple act of juicing will take your physical performance to another level. Eight ounces of vegetable juice a day is the simplest, most cost-effective and powerful way to boost your health nutritionally. The best part is that even if you don't eat all of your veggies every day, you can just drink them in five minutes!

This simple habit has increased my athletic performance almost as much as anything I've done. Why? The breadth and depth of nutrients you get in a glass of pure, fresh vegetable juice is beyond compare: it is loaded with super-healthy bioflavonoids, antioxidants, and phytonutrients. In fact, freshly prepared vegetable juices are so healthy that when you have a tall glass, if you pay close attention to your body, you can *feel* its healthful effects almost immediately.

Your homemade juices should be 80 percent vegetables and 20 percent fruit, which keeps them lower on the glycemic index (see appendix B). Excellent foods for juicing are celery, apples, carrots, spinach, cucumber, ginger, and kale. Experiment with different vegetables until you find the perfect recipe.

~~~~~~

ACTION ITEM

Research a few juicers and purchase one this month. The most reliable and cost-effective juicer I've used is the *Juiceman II*.

38. Once a Week, Leave the Devices at Home

I am a gadget nut, and it drives my fiancée mad. If a new product comes out, I must have it. You say it's more expensive and offers absolutely nothing new or better? No matter. I still must have it. This applies to my training as well, but it can get out of hand: I've been known to leave the house looking like Robocop, wearing a heart monitor, two stopwatches, lactate analyzer, MP3 player, full body suit, and dark sunglasses!

While some exercise gadgets facilitate better fitness results, they can also disconnect your mind from your body during exercise. As we've learned, music is an effective training tool (tip #32), but you tend to exercise to the beat of your music as opposed to the beat of your body. On a spiritual level, gadgets can disconnect you from the special moments that are often hidden during exercise. I know that when I've got the Chemical Brothers blaring in my ears, I do not notice anything except my performance.

That is one reason why runners are purists: shoes, socks, shorts, and a shirt. Pretty minimalist, but some Olympic runners feel that training with the bare minimum of equipment liberates them, physically and emotionally, and frees them up for even better performances.

~~~~~~

ACTION ITEM

Once this week, leave all the gadgets at home and be spontaneous in a work-out. This is about relinquishing control of your pace to your body. Let your body dictate the pace and rhythm of your workout.

39. When You're Unmotivated to Exercise, Begin for Five Minutes, Then Decide

~~~~~~

Our greatest battles are those with our own minds.

—FRANK JAMESON, POET

One of the big stumbling blocks to achieving higher levels of fitness is staying motivated. If you've done your homework and identified your ends motivations (tip #2), it's just a matter of overcoming that superficial, yet dangerous, mental debate each day. Before many exercise sessions, we all go through that debate:

Your Mind: *Should I really do this? I'm exhausted.*

You: *Oh, come on. You love running, and you are getting fitter by the day!*

Your Mind: *Look at that, it's about to rain. Let's hit the road first thing tomorrow.*

You: *Great. What's on television?*

Almost invariably, if you go too deeply into the mental debate about whether or not to exercise, your mind will convince you not to work out. One reason the world's best athletes get out the door each day is that they avoid this debate altogether. Another answer is to implement the five-minute rule. Many Olympic champions use this simple strategy to get out the door every morning.

The majority of the time, our minds convince us to skip exercise when in fact our bodies are quite ready for the workout. I've had my best workouts when I ignored my mind even as it insisted my body was tired. The best way to get motivated is to take action. Just five minutes: that's all you must commit to. Give yourself the very real option to turn around. Nine times out of ten you will end up doing your entire workout.

If you're incredibly unmotivated, here's a trick I learned from a professional track athlete: she called it "the get dressed slowly method" (GDSM). This is how it's done: You've just come home from work. You're exhausted. The last thing you want to do is go running. Okay, I'm with you. You don't need to do anything. Just slip off your work shirt and put on a running shirt.

That's it! Nothing more. Walk around your house with your running shirt on. Have some water, read a magazine, and ten minutes later . . . get your running shorts on. Sit on the couch for a few minutes and, without thought, slide on your running shoes. Relax, watch a little TV, then when the next commercial comes on, get up and walk right out the front door. You won. Your mind didn't even catch on to what was happening. Now that you're out the door, your body will take over from here.

40. Run Like the Kenyans

The Kenyan runners are the best in the world. How do these tranquil people from a tiny nation dominate the sport of running worldwide? Much of it has to do with genetics, running great lengths as children, and living in a country that treasures its runners. But there's something bigger—something we can all learn from the Kenyans: *they increase their composure as the intensity heightens.*

Think about that for a moment. If you could learn to relax as your stress levels increase, can you imagine how much more in control you'd be during exercise and in daily life? When the Kenyans are deep into a marathon and the heat is really on, they look entirely composed. I learned more about this powerful technique while running with the Kenyan runners in Lanzarote, a small island off the coast of Morocco.

I decided to train with the Kenyans in order to bring my running to the highest possible level (tip #28). For the first five days I was an outsider, and the

Kenyans did little to help me through the mind-numbingly difficult workouts. They ran, and if I fell behind, tough luck. It wasn't until the sixth day of training that they opened up and revealed their secrets about athletic performance. What took them hundreds of thousands of miles and generations to learn, I had to *earn*. And to do that, I had to run with them. Twenty-two miles a day. In the hills. And *fast*.

In the middle of a particularly tough climb, I began to heave from the pain of the effort. I remember the pain running so deep, my eyes began to cross. One of the Kenyans leaned over and said: "As it gets harder, you need to get easier." As the climb continued, I tried to divert some energy from my legs to my brain to think about this. I was in so much more pain than the Kenyans, and it wasn't because they were that much fitter than me. It was almost as if my mind was "creating" more pain and effort than there really was. Have you ever done that? You're doing something that's stressful, like paying bills, and your mind makes the process *feel* a whole lot worse than it is. My experience with the Kenyans was the physical equivalent of paying bills. I was getting far more stressed out than I needed to be.

So during this particular run, I took a few deep breaths, centered myself, wiped the "perception of pain" from my mind, and immediately felt a comforting ease sweep over my body. Amazingly, my heart rate dropped, my stride lengthened, and I caught the faster runners. I was running like the Kenyans, and it was the most important lesson I had ever learned about performance.

~~~~~~

ACTION ITEM

We have a tendency to make things more complex and difficult than they really are. Try not to. When things get stressful during exercise or in daily life, learn to put forth great effort with a calm, loose body. Maintain your mental composure. If you approach your workouts and your daily life just as the Kenyans run, by relaxing as you increase the effort, your human performance will soar.

41. Treat Workouts Like Important Appointments

The first wealth is health.
—RALPH WALDO EMERSON, WRITER (1803–1882)

If health is our number one priority, why do we relegate exercise to the end of our to-do lists? I suspect it's because we can't directly feel the damage done when we neglect our bodies from missing just one workout. Well, I can assure you: your body is keeping score. And someday it'll demand payment. With interest.

This is not about turning your workouts into work. As we learned in tip #19, exercise is meant to be play, not work. This speaks to giving more reverence to your *workout time*. There are certain things in your life that you will not miss: for example, time with your children. Exercise is your fountain of youth, and it deserves a higher priority in your life. Often we fail to make firm appointments with ourselves for the things most important in our lives. Have a look at your daily planner. Does this week include solitary time alone? With your spouse? With your children? Does it include exercise time? If so, you are a power prioritizer. Our planners should physically reflect what is most important to us—and fitness should be at the top of our list.

~~~~~~

ACTION ITEM

Write your exercise sessions (from tip #4) into your daily planner, your PalmPilot, and your Outlook Calendar. Assign a "high priority" to those workouts and don't let anybody take that time from you.

42. Break Down Long Workouts into Simple, Bite-Size Morsels

Ann Trason has won the Western States one-hundred-mile running race a record ten times—steamrolling many of the top men along the way. Her secret is how she *sees* the race. Most competitors view it as a one-hundred-mile run and naturally become overwhelmed by its magnitude. Ann breaks down the race into small, "easily digestible segments." In this way, her race is far less daunting and gives her simple checkpoints on which to focus. Like most champion athletes, Ann begins the race with one step—her best step—then takes another and another, stringing together single steps that result in a one-hundred-mile triumph. Top athletes face long, painful races this way. If you view long, difficult tasks in this way, you will perform far better and with greater ease.

In your next workout or athletic event, string together segments of doing your best, and before you know it you have a full, uninterrupted masterpiece of your best effort. Think in terms of small chunks of distance or time: five-minute segments or two-kilometer increments, rather than the whole time or distance. You'll find that this approach keeps you focused on the present and on doing your best each step of the way. The next time you perform a long task in life, apply this powerfully effective technique as well.

43. Work Out with the One You Love

~~~~~~

Few of us lie on our deathbed and lament: "I wish I'd spent more time in the office." The irony is that we seem to gain our clearest perspective when we lose the ability to change our lives. People who have faced great personal tragedy or people at the end of their lives invariably point to not having spent enough time with, or said enough loving words to, the people they care about most. It is important to accept the practical necessities of life (such as work, traffic, laundry), but it is equally important to address our emotional needs that so often go unfulfilled. Daily exercise provides a perfect way to fulfill those needs.

Of the over ten thousand workouts I've done, the most rewarding ones are the easy runs alongside my fiancée on her mountain bike across the trails of Mt. Tamalpais. (Since I'm a little faster than she is, she rides her mountain bike as I run. Most top athletes train with others by similarly "evening the odds.")

Exercising with someone you care about can be a deeply bonding experience. Decide which activity you want to do together and schedule regular workouts together—*no excuses*. Make this an ironclad commitment to one another. Thanks to today's hectic lifestyle, people advocate "quality over quantity" in relationships. That's a copout. If you care deeply about someone, you must have lots of *quantity* to deepen the *quality* of that relationship. Exercise provides the ideal time each day to do that.

44. Eat Well, Exercise Smart

Long-term health or fitness success cannot be bought; it comes from your ironclad decision to make incremental and important lifestyle changes. This is especially true these days, when more than ever you must be skeptical of hyped weight loss products or machines. Ninety percent simply do not deliver what they promise, because they are not geared to our passion for exercise. They are designed to be sold in mass quantities. Be particularly skeptical of fad diets. Fad diets are precisely that, fads. It's just a matter of time before they are "out of style." The most timeless nutritional strategy is to stick with food that gives you long-term energy and a positive frame of mind. Period.

When tempted to buy another fitness product or buy into another nutrition fad, turn yourself instead to smarter exercise and better nutrition. This will produce far better (and less expensive) results, every time. Empower yourself, not the fitness industry.

45. Turn Fear into Confidence

A hero is no braver than an ordinary man, but he is braver five minutes longer.

—RALPH WALDO EMERSON, WRITER (1803–1882)

Emerson was right on the money. When you look at the world's best athletes before competitions, it looks as if their steely confidence runs to the core. Not entirely true. Many of these people are hiding fear, anxiety, and enormous stress. They've simply mastered these emotions and learned to channel them into positive action (tip #25). You can learn to transform your fear into confidence as well. It's all based on your physiology.

While fear can undermine almost everything we do, confidence can empower us to do almost anything. There are precise, simple techniques champion athletes use to transform their fear immediately into a winning confidence—that is what separates them from the field. Two of the simplest, most powerful techniques are "anchoring" and "acting."

Anchoring is an effective skill that you can learn quite easily. It involves reconnecting to past successes. You literally relive the experience in rich detail: how determined and strong you were, how confident you felt. As you anchor yourself to those feelings of successful past events, your body begins to take on a new confidence in the present. The fastest way to resurrect those feelings is to refer to your success journal (tip #7).

Acting is the other technique top athletes use to transform fear into confidence. As I mentioned, at the start of many races top athletes don't always feel ready or confident, but the best ones can summon positive emotions on command. You can, too, and this can be a powerful ally in any stressful situation. Late in races, when pain reaches a crescendo, the best athletes look the most composed. Their secret is simple: They fake it. They act as if they feel fantastic, and they start believing it. Studies have shown that when people *pretend* to feel a certain way, beginning with something as small as a smile, it elicits profound physical changes throughout the body. In a very physical sense, motion determines emotion, which illustrates the enormous potential of a strong mind-body connection.

ACTION ITEM

The next time you find yourself in a fearful or difficult situation, act as if you are supremely confident. Take a deep breath, assume a power position—both feet planted firmly on the ground, shoulders back, head up—and smile. If you can positively influence your mood on command, you've gone a long way to controlling every life situation, which is exactly what shapes good athletes into champions.

46. "Bad Days" Are a Good Sign

~~~~~~

The human body undergoes significant changes each day: fluctuating moods, varying levels of hydration, and powerful hormonal shifts. We often feel those effects in our workouts: one day we're floating through our exercise effortlessly, the next we feel as if we're running through cotton.

The first thing to realize is that having off days in workouts is completely normal. The world's best athletes have them at least twice a week. In fact, "off days" are a good sign—your body is telling you it's time to take it easy or to rest. All you have to do is act on those signals.

Many of us fight our bodies when they don't respond to our commands during exercise. We get progressively more frustrated during the workout. But the fact may be that your body simply isn't ready to work out that day. There are two things you can do on an "off day": You can turn right around and head home. That's perfectly okay. I've seen top swimmers, ten minutes into a session, just jump out of the pool and call it quits. At that time, their bodies are not receptive to training, and exercising would be detrimental to their long-term progress.

The other option is to just let go of your physical expectations and simply "smooth through" the session. I've actually had my best workouts when I relinquished all performance goals and just trained entirely on feel.

We also get discouraged when we have one, two, or three bad workouts in a row. Don't. If the best athletes in the world have poor workout days regularly, you should expect them, too. The worst thing you can do is quit your program because of a bad week.

~~~~~~

ACTION ITEM

When you're not feeling good during a workout, just ease through it. Don't fight your body. There is a great lesson in learning to let go of expectation and accept what simply "is."

47. Meditate in Motion

~~~~~~

Mark Allen, the greatest triathlete ever, called exercise and athletic competition "a meditation in motion." Interesting statement from a man nick-named "the Grip," a man who raced for blood. Allen was notorious for maintaining almost perfect mental equanimity during even the most intense physical efforts.

When most of us think of meditation, we picture someone sitting alone, motionless in a quiet room, with incense burning. I'm a big fan of getting things done while in motion, particularly during exercise, and I suggest you learn to meditate while you are working out. The best part of meditating in motion is that you get all the mental benefits of meditation and all the physical benefits of aerobic exercise.

I learned how to meditate in motion from a professional swimmer. The first and most important step is to choose a peaceful setting in which to exercise (tip #31). When you're out there, clear your thoughts (tip #18) and be present in the moment (tip #21). The idea is to remain as mentally relaxed as possible, and the best way to do that is to focus entirely on your breathing. After about ten minutes of focusing on the soothing rhythm of your breath, you will naturally enter progressively deeper meditative states. Invariably you will get distracted by thoughts or by your surroundings; just move those distractions aside as they come up and get back to your breathing. Keep these workouts at a steady, aerobic pace.

ACTION ITEM

Allocate one workout sometime over the next two weeks as a "meditative session." This doesn't mean you can't perform out there, just maintain a mental calm while your body is active. This "duality" of mind and body during exercise can be a very exciting and rewarding experience.

48. Never Miss a Chance to Risk Being Great

Risk can be terrifying. Inherent in that word is the very real chance of public failure and humiliation. We become so afraid of looking bad that we avoid things we know we should try. The only way to achieve greatness is to operate well outside of our comfort zone, to take calculated risks.

I've had hundreds of failures in my career, but the shining victories more than make up for those failures. Top athletes seize every chance they get to be great. You can, too, but first you must come to terms with fear of failure.

As we will learn in the next tip, failure is nothing more than education. It is how we grow. It means we're moving outside of our realm of understanding, and to me, that is pretty courageous. I learned a profound lesson about risk and failure while on a training run in France. One of their top professional cyclists said to me: "Americans are deathly afraid of risk. So afraid, they avoid doing things they want to do! Here, we see failure as part of success. It motivates us. It means we're learning and growing. It excites and inspires us."

The best way to deal with failure is with humor. I've learned to smile at every single one of my mistakes—I learn from them, but I smile at them. Part of the reason I smile is that I'm so proud I was willing to move outside of my comfort zone.

~~~~~~

ACTION ITEM

When you redefine failure as education, you will begin to try new things—just as you did as a child. When we take a risk and push a little further, our confidence soars. So it's time to go . . . bungee jumping. Seriously. Do something that scares the hell out of you. This is the kind of suggestion that you must take action on immediately, today. Call a bungee jumping or skydiving company right now and sign up. You can do it.

49. Make Lots of Mistakes

The credit belongs to those who are actually in the arena, who strive valiantly; who know the great enthusiasm, the great devotions, and spend themselves in a worthy cause; who at the best, know the triumph of high achievement; and who at the worst, if they fail, fail while daring greatly, so that their place shall never be with those cold and timid souls who know neither victory or defeat.

—THEODORE ROOSEVELT, TWENTY-SIXTH PRESIDENT OF THE UNITED STATES
   (1858–1919)

As children, we made mistakes constantly. When we learned to ride a bike, we fell down twenty-two times, and we didn't care. We kept getting back up until we were streaming down the road on that bike . . . without a clue as to how to stop. Stopping would be learned soon enough. That complete willingness to make mistakes in order to learn something new and exciting is one reason children learn at such a wonderfully fast rate. Somewhere along the line, we were "taught" that mistakes were bad. In fact, we developed such an aversion to making mistakes that some of us simply stopped trying new things. That is such a shame. I can tell you, the world's best athletes never, ever stop trying new things. Making lots of mistakes is how world records are broken.

Here's a little-known fact about Michael Jordan: His lifetime field goal percentage is 49.6 percent. One of the most revered athletes in history failed more than he has succeeded. The thing is this: *He never stopped shooting.* If you make a mistake, it means you're stretching your limits. That's good. You're "actually in the arena," striving valiantly; knowing the great enthusiasm! You should never, ever feel bad about that.

~~~~~~

ACTION ITEM

This week try a new sport and stretch your limits. Resolve beforehand that if you make a couple of well-intentioned mistakes, you will laugh at yourself and smooth right through them. Embrace the learning process just as you did when you were a child. Mistakes can be pretty painless if we shift our perspective a little and stop taking ourselves so seriously.

50. No Guilt—Seriously, No Guilt

Guilt may very well be the most useless emotion there is. Think about it for a moment: you decide to do something, and afterward you realize it wasn't a good decision, so you get mired in guilt. Meanwhile, nothing is getting done. You're in no-man's-land. Guilt is a disempowering, problem-centric emotion. And it has no place in a life filled with passion and performance.

Champion athletes have zero guilt about missing exercise. If they miss a workout, they always make the best of the situation by doing something fun or productive or by letting that missed session strengthen their resolve for the next workout. At some point, we've all felt guilty about missing a workout. I say either do the workout and feel great about it, or skip it and feel equally great. The worst part about guilt is that it keeps us from enjoying the fact that we just got to skip a workout!

This is a big reason people quit new fitness programs. They miss one or two or even ten workouts, and they decide "it's no longer worth it." Wrong! You can get back to your fitness at any moment, whether it's after one day or one year. People often say to me: "I began a great new fitness program and stuck to it for three weeks. Then I quit. I failed." My response is: "Are you crazy?" Three weeks of exercise is fantastic. You just improved your life by twenty-one days! View your fitness within the context of your entire life. If you live thirty-five thousand days, the more of those days that include exercise, the better your life will be. Adopting this broader perspective will allay the guilt you feel when you miss workouts in the short term.

ACTION ITEM

Remove guilt from your emotional catalog. That's it, gone. If you can't let go of guilt entirely, commit to at least never, ever feeling guilt about your fitness again. The next time you skip a workout, do so without remorse. Make the most of that free time and simply commit to getting right back to business the next day. That's what the champions do.

51. Replace Coffee with Green Tea

I'm a green tea freak. Before every key workout, big competition, or important meeting, I drink a giant jar of loose-leaf green tea. It looks like a science project, but it's high-horsepower fuel. Green tea—and I'm talking about the authentic loose-leaf stuff—is one of the most powerful substances on the planet. It has one of the highest concentrations of antioxidants of any food or beverage. Green tea is a mainstay of the Japanese diet, which may account for their remarkably low incidences of cancer.

Most of us have a love affair with coffee, but I regret to say that coffee is not the healthiest thing for your body. In fact, some research has shown that there are over two hundred mild "toxins" in coffee. I'm not certain about that, but I do know that green tea is a much better alternative. It has more antioxidants and none of the acidity, and it provides the same swift mental kick as coffee.

ACTION ITEM

I know it's tough, but this week try to replace your coffee with green tea. You'll find the loose-leaf variety located in the "bins" of your favorite health food store. Sencha green tea is my personal favorite. Greet each morning with a tall glass of green tea and you will experience a greater feeling of health and mental clarity.

52. Don't Let Others Determine Your Limits—Define Your Own

~~~~~~

After Fred Astaire's first screen test, the evaluating memo read: "Can't act. Slightly bald. Can dance a little."

Who were these people? Were they blind? As you know by now, I am not a big fan of negative critics. Unfortunately, much of the time we allow others to define our limits. For some strange reason, it's easier to hear the negative things about ourselves than to accept the positive ones. Why is that? Whatever the reason, there are things you can do to remain immune to the nonsensical ramblings of negative critics.

"Critics" who tear down our confidence and fill us with self-doubt constantly bombard athletes. It's almost as if they are waiting for us to fail. As a survival mechanism, champions have developed precise ways to stay immune to their negativity. One technique is to simply not give negative critics the same respect you would give normal people. Some of the top baseball and football players do this. The extreme example is Mike Ditka, the former coach of the Chicago Bears. Have you ever seen Mike Ditka talk to a reporter? This is a guy who knows how to handle skeptics. He responds to negative, nonconstructive criticism with zero tolerance. We're all sensitive about our bodies and our fitness. That is why we are particularly susceptible to criticism in these areas.

Learn to recognize when others try to define our limits—and defy them.

53. Sign Up for a Race and Pay Now

The race is a simple, uncomplicated confrontation with myself.
—GEORGE SHEEHAN, M.D., AUTHOR, *RUNNING & BEING* (1998)

Those of you who have competed in an organized event know what a transforming experience it can be. Its effects can last a lifetime and affect every area of your life. There is no doubt that athletic competition will show you that you are capable of far more than you know, because it will, in the most tangible sense, expand your perceived limits. Steve Prefontaine, one of the best competitors of all time, saw a race not so much as a competition against other people, but as a test to see how far the human heart can go. This is what participating in an athletic event is all about.

Sign up for a race six to eight weeks away and pay now. This will create a time-based deadline to keep you motivated and locked on your fitness goal. You don't need to win the race, just go out and push yourself beyond what you thought was possible. Seize the moment. There is a point in any competition where you reach your limit. Some people decide to quit, and others say: "I can do this." Choose the latter. The pleasure at the finish will surpass all the pain you felt. In fact, the harder you try and the more fear you overcome, the greater your satisfaction. Your pain will wash away into euphoria when you have given your all. After an effort like this, you will feel very different about yourself.

54. Eat Good Fats

~~~~~~

As a nation, we've been driven to completely fear dietary fats. Ironic, isn't it, that at a time when we've never eaten less fat, we're fatter than ever? The secret is not avoiding fat altogether; it's about shunning *bad* fats. Hydrogenated fats (those found in cookies, crackers, and cakes) and saturated fats (butter, fatty meats, and so on) are the real culprits.

Small amounts of "quality fats," on the other hand, are absolutely essential to good health. They restore proper hormonal balance; they are an extremely powerful source of fuel during exercise; and they satisfy you. Eating fat can actually result in overall lower consumption of calories. Take this example: Two plain bagels total 600 calories. One bagel with some low-fat cream cheese is only 450 calories. Which one makes you feel more satisfied? See how adding quality fat to foods can help you lose weight and enjoy eating more?

Your diet should consist of 15–20 percent quality fats: extra-virgin olive oil, avocado, flax oil, peanut butter, and fish oil. Don't fear fats; they are important to enjoying your food and essential to maintaining your good health.

55. Active Rest Is Dynamic Recovery

Active rest is an integral part of every full-time athlete's life. In fact, it's what takes the most time. For me, it's not the thirty hours a week of training I think about, it's the time I must spend restoring my body. Top endurance athletes have discovered ways to actually "accelerate" the recovery process, because it is so vital to their livelihoods: the quicker you can recover, the quicker you can get out for the next workout—while your competition is still convalescing!

That's why steroids are so effective. Essentially, they reduce that "time to recovery" period to almost zilch—the moment you complete a workout, you're ready for the next one. But true champions, those who beat the cheats, have shown that intelligent training coupled with "active rest" is more powerful than any drug, and far healthier as well. You can use the following simple techniques to accelerate the recovery process from your workouts and your work:

➤ Take a hot bath and elevate your legs for five minutes afterward. This is a favorite among top cyclists because it provides such effective recovery for your legs by "flushing out" the waste products that build up in your legs from being on your feet all day. Add some essential oils or sea salts to your baths.
➤ Take an easy walk or a relaxed swim. Don't underestimate the healing benefits of easy exercise. These are excellent recovery methods, since you are pumping blood through your body without stressing it.
➤ Treat yourself to the awesome healing properties of a high-quality one-hour massage, particularly after tough workouts or workdays. This is not a luxury. Sometimes it's a necessity. My mom views bodywork as a "utility bill" that she must pay each month. I love that.
➤ Hyperhydrate for one day. Most of us are chronically dehydrated, and this is a powerful way to reestablish a healthy homeostatic balance in your body. Drink at least twenty 8-ounce glasses of water for one day. Yes, you will be

peeing every hour, but the recuperative benefits from this process are well worth the extra trips to the bathroom.

➤ Explore hot-cold hydrotherapy. This is fantastic for boosting your immunity. Take a hot bath for five minutes, then a cold shower for thirty seconds. Repeat this process three times, then lie down in a quiet, dark room for ten minutes. You will feel relaxed and fantastic.

56. Measure Your Progress with Benchmark Workouts

That which is measured, improves.

—ANONYMOUS

Improving at something motivates us to do it more. Benchmark workouts are the best way to gauge your fitness progress and to stay motivated to exercise over the long term.

Benchmark workouts can prevent overtraining and predict oncoming illness. Once you establish a baseline of fitness, a workout that falls below that is usually a sign of bad things to come: you need to either rest, rework your nutrition, or adjust your training schedule. As you do more of these sessions, you will develop a deeper body awareness. You will learn how to move with greater efficiency, strength, and grace. This will work wonders on your passion and performance.

Benchmark sessions can help you determine technical modifications to and the overall effectiveness of your training programs. For example, on a cycling benchmark, I learned that raising my seat just one-half inch bettered my time by 3 percent. More broadly, by looking at my benchmark workouts, I discovered that five days per week of exercise was far more beneficial than four.

Most important, these sessions build your confidence. When your workout shows good numbers, it reflects positively on your rest, exercise, and nutrition. The best athletes in the world continue to improve because they are constantly checking their progress with benchmark workouts. You should, too.

ACTION ITEM

Establish your baseline aerobic fitness. After a ten-to-fifteen minute warm-up, cover a fixed distance—walk, run, cycle, or swim—at a specific heart rate and compare your times over the weeks. A fitter body will go faster at the same heart rate. Be sure to perform your benchmark workouts on the same course every time. Note: These workouts are almost impossible to perform without the use of a heart rate monitor (tip #23), which will indicate exactly how hard you are working.

57. Eat Fat and Protein Before Workouts, Carbohydrates and Sugar After

~~~~~~

This simple strategy will make a real improvement in the quality of your workouts. What and when you eat before exercise has a profound impact on the quality of that workout. It's all about insulin and blood sugar. Different "nutrition experts" have written countless books on this subject and packaged it in all sorts of fancy ways, but the message is the same: Keep your insulin as steady as possible, particularly before and during exercise, and you will be healthier, happier, and fitter.

There is no doubt that you will have your best workouts when your insulin is steady. Sugar and carbohydrates elevate insulin, which prevents your body from using body fat as fuel during exercise and makes you feel lethargic during exercise. Protein and fats elicit less of an insulin response and should be consumed before exercise.

For the thirty to sixty minutes after completing a workout, your body is most receptive to absorbing nutrients. Within that window of time, it's important to eat a good balance of protein and carbos, with something sweet if you went particularly hard. After tough workouts, you'll see some of the world's best athletes eating all sorts of naughty foods—candy bars, sodas, even ice cream. My personal favorite is a Snickers bar after interval sessions, because eating sugar after strenuous workouts will actually help your body more quickly resynthesize the glycogen it used. In addition, having sugary foods after workouts will do far less damage to you than if you eat them at any other time of day.

~~~~~~

ACTION ITEM

This week, eat protein and quality fats before your workout and sugar and carbohydrates after exercise. For example, a peanut butter sandwich before and a banana after. Observe how that makes you feel during workouts and in the hours and days following strenuous exercise.

58. Smooth Out Life's Transitions

Transitions are a major part of life. We are constantly moving between one project and the next. One of life's toughest transitions is between work and workouts. Most people are mentally and physically drained from work, which leaves very little energy for exercise. The secret is to master the art of transitions.

Transitions are a major part of my sport, triathlon. Moving among three very different sports with different physiological and psychological demands is something that has taken me years to master. I learned that how I rode the bike portion determined, in large part, how I ran.

The secret to mastering the transition from your work to your workouts lies in how you treat yourself *at work*. If you keep your stress levels down, graze well, and drink enough water throughout the day, you will leave work fresher and you will have more energy to exercise in the evening.

In addition to the above strategy, a physical, symbolic transition will sometimes help move you from the mental demands of work to the physical demands of exercise. Take a hot shower before evening workouts. It will wash away fatigue from your workday and allow a smoother transition to exercise.

59. In Bed by Ten

I discovered that the advice my mom always gave me is the mantra of every top athlete around the globe. You may think there is simply no way you can be in bed by ten o'clock on a consistent basis. I'm here to say you can. You may have to rearrange your life a little, but the effects from this one tip will lead to a much higher quality of life: more productivity at work, improved moods, increased energy, even a longer life. I'm willing to bet you could use a bit more high-quality sleep. Many of us are chronically sleep deprived, which manifests itself in irritability, fatigue, and diminished mental clarity. As our calendars have grown fuller, our sleep has been shortened.

ACTION ITEM

The key to success with this strategy is to be unwavering in your commitment to it. Be in bed by ten o'clock every night for one week. Set your watch for nine-thirty and begin preparing for bed at that time. You may feel guilty, as if you shouldn't be going to bed that early. Let that feeling go. Your sleep will absolutely make you a far more productive and happy human being, and you should not feel guilty about that.

After the week is done, determine if the benefits of getting to bed earlier are worth the sacrifice. I think you'll find, as the majority of champion athletes have found, that they are.

60. Once a Month, Be Well Rested and Give Your All in a Workout

~~~~~~

There is only one real failure in life that is possible, and that is not to be true to the best we know.

—FREDERICK FARRAR, WRITER/EDUCATOR (1831–1903)

"Breakthrough sessions" are one of the best ways to reach a new level of athletic performance and a higher level of self-confidence. These sessions are all about forging your passion into physical performance. They are the cornerstones of every great athlete's training program. In a breakthrough session, you physically exceed anything you've done before in that activity.

Perhaps the most important benefit of these exciting workouts is that they instantly and profoundly reveal your true inner strength—you learn what you've really got in you, mentally and physically. When you discover the real power that lies within you, how much further you can push, you reset your level of self-esteem to maximum.

~~~~~~

It's important to be mentally and physically prepared for these workouts. Rest and eat well in the two days before your breakthrough session. (Note: In order to avoid injury, you should do breakthrough sessions only if you've got at least six weeks of consistent [three-plus days per week] aerobic conditioning under your belt.)

Get excited about this workout. You are about to break through to a new level of passion and performance! Begin the session with a thorough warm-up. You may want to stretch for a few minutes after the warm-up as well. For the next five minutes, clear your mind, fill yourself with confidence, and visualize your body as a strong, powerful machine. When you are ready for the breakthrough portion, take a deep breath and let it fly. The breakthrough portion of your workout need not last longer than a couple of minutes. The idea is to push beyond what you previously thought was possible—to redefine your limits. Let's use a forty-minute run as an example: You warm up gradually over the first ten minutes. Then you may do ten minutes of nice, steady running at 70 percent of your maximum heart rate—a pace that feels comfortable but challenging. Follow this with an easy three-to-five-minute walk to recharge your mind and body as you mentally center yourself for the "breakthrough portion" of the workout. For two minutes, you run faster, stronger, or better than you ever have. It need not be the *fastest* you've ever run, just the *best*—the most focused, relaxed, confident, whatever you want to develop that day. Since exercise is meant to empower your life just as much as it boosts your fitness, view your breakthrough workouts as a physical, tangible way to "break through" to new levels of performance, fitness, confidence, and self-esteem. When you finish the workout, let the passion of a breakthrough performance course through your body. Burn that feeling into your mind.

Be sure to record these workouts in your success journal (tip #7). Your breakthrough sessions will become invaluable, cherished experiences to you.

61. No Home Exercise Gadget Can Beat Simple Push-Ups and Sit-Ups

I'm not going to get away with this one. The exercise machine manufacturers will surely exact their wrath. But come on, aren't these machines getting a little ridiculous? Most of them do little for our long-term fitness and end up under the bed or drying wet clothes anyway.

Physiologically there is very little difference between the benefits you would derive from any of the popular home exercise machines and those from a good, steady helping of push-ups and sit-ups.

This strategy is as ideological as it is pragmatic in that we need to move *away from* paying other people to help us achieve our fitness goals and rely more on ourselves. We are so much more powerful than those people want us to think we are.

ACTION ITEM

Stop spending money on exercise machines. If you want to begin a home exercise routine, simply do push-ups and sit-ups. To add excitement to those workouts, play music that really motivates you (tip #32). If you really must buy exercise equipment, buy a set of used dumbbells at a secondhand store. You'll save money and time, and you'll get the same benefit you would from an expensive home exercise machine.

62. Chocolate Heals

~~~~~~

I'm a chocoholic. I got it from my mom, who is legendary for her addiction to chocolate. Easter, with its rich supply of chocolate bunnies, was her favorite holiday.

My mom ate chocolate because it provided her with a deep, soothing comfort. The key was that she was very judicious about it—limiting her indulgences to only once a week. Some Native Americans view chocolate as a "healer," because it tastes so good. Can you imagine? The food tastes so good that it produces healing chemicals in the body. You should eat food that soothes you on a regular but infrequent basis. Being "bad" (tip #15) once in a while is vital to your long-term mental health.

Let the deprivation thing go. Just use the tips in this book to exercise smarter and eat better. If you want chocolate once in a while, eat it. And savor every bite.

63. Recognize and Act on Stress Before It Becomes Part of You

Physical and mental stress drains the passion from our lives, compromises our health, and can cost us a lot of time and money. Some people wear the physical signs of stress on their faces—the stress has become part of who they are. And if it shows on the outside, it's eating them up on the inside. This is not what you want, and it's easy to ensure it doesn't happen to you.

While many of us treat stress symptomatically with drugs only when it interferes with daily life, the real key is to prevent stress from happening altogether. Top athletes are masters of diverting mental and physical stress before it hits. They do this by recognizing the very early signs of stress and resolving that stress before it becomes problematic.

Developing a deeper body sensitivity will allow you to recognize *where* the stress is coming from and how deeply it is affecting you. When you know that, you must act on those early warning signals. Early detection is great, but early *action* is the key.

When you feel stress coming on, there are two simple things top athletes do that you can do to help reduce or eliminate the stress almost completely:

1. Breathe through your nose. This instantly engages the parasympathetic (relaxation) response and will bring instant physical relief from stress. The next tip covers this powerful technique in greater detail.

2. Immediately pull back physically and mentally. Champion athletes do this before every competition with great success; that is why you see athletes sitting in the middle of nowhere before races. Stress is insidious, building in you imperceptibly until you lose control of it. When you feel your heart rate or blood pressure rise, it's time, right then and there, to move to another physical location and to clear your head. Getting outdoors is best. Take a few moments to center yourself, then come back to the situation.

You will gain more control over your life when you pay more attention to your emotions throughout the day and learn to quickly resolve negative feelings.

64. Breathe Through Your Nose

~~~~~~

Catch any top athlete right before the start of a major competition and you will see three things: a total relaxed focus; a calm, loose body; and deep breathing in through the nose and out of the mouth.

As you learned in the previous tip, a simple way to deal with stress in one swift motion is breathing through your nose. Deep, diaphragmatic breathing is what elite athletes use to control pre-event tension, and this simple, effortless, highly effective skill will work for you in most stressful situations.

Breathing through your nose engages the parasympathetic, or relaxation, response. Your blood pressure and heart rates go down, and you begin to feel more relaxed and positive. Conversely, shallow breathing, or "panting" with your upper chest, triggers your "fight or flight" response, and that increases your stress level.

Breathing through your nose while at rest is excellent for stress reduction. Breathe through your nose *during exercise* and your workouts will reach another level. I remember watching the 4x400 relay at the 1996 Olympics. The final U.S. runner, Anthuan Maybank, had just a two-meter lead on Britain's Roger Black, the Olympic silver medallist, at four hundred meters. The U.S. runner was breathing through his nose the entire time . . . in one of the most anaerobic events there is. He was far more composed than Black, and his confidence seemed to build through the four hundred meters. By the end, he was in complete mental and physical control. Black was a wreck.

To enter "the performance zone" during exercise, focus on breathing in through your nose and out through your mouth. Focus actively on the exhalation and let the inhalation "just happen." (If you have trouble breathing through your nose, Breathe Rights are not simply a fashion statement, they really do work well.) Breathe Rights are small strips you place on your nose to increase air flow. You may have seen them on the noses of NFL players, most notably Jerry Rice of the 49'ers.

Try three "diaphragmatic breaths" right now. Sit in a comfortable position and close your eyes. Inhale deeply through your nose, counting to ten. Go deep, and expand your belly, not your chest. Go all the way to the deep recesses of your lungs and tune in to the positive changes in your body. Hold it for three seconds and ease the air out for a count of five. As you exhale, visualize the stress melting off your body. Now, *that's* a breath.

65. If You've Lost the Passion for Your Sport or Exercise, Switch Sports

~~~~~~

What rule states that you have to stick with one exercise or sport for the rest of your life? Grinding through a rigid, one-dimensional fitness program will do little for your passion or your performance. Remember, our physical activity is meant to *add* passion to our lives. This must always, always be the goal of exercise.

A common misconception about exercise is that it must be regimented, almost devoid of enjoyment. Untrue! Anything that gets your heart humming along in the right heart zones (tip #24) is considered aerobic exercise. Basketball, tennis, and hiking are all equally beneficial to your aerobic system.

If you've grown tired of your exercise, seize the moment, act on your childlike passion, and pick another sport. My friend Walter Lightner is a perfect example of this. He runs, bikes, and swims constantly. He's also acutely aware of how much exercise feeds his soul. Last winter Walter lost the passion for his exercise—he had cycled, swum, and run one time too many. One day, while driving, he saw a row of batting cages gleaming from off the highway. Baseball was Walter's favorite sport as a child. So right there, without hesitation, he pulled off the freeway and walked straight into the batting cages.

Eighty quarters, two hours, and 160 balls later, Walter's arms were so sore that he could barely lift them. His body was exhausted, but his exercise passion was revitalized! And by the way, he had just burned through three thousand calories and finished an incredible strength session. That is the feeling you want to capture as often as possible in your exercise, and if it means switching sports more often, then do it. It may not be practical to switch sports constantly. The idea is to keep an exciting amount of variety in your fitness program and to not be afraid to try new things.

66. The Final Word on Great Abdominals

A high-performance tummy will lead to great passion and improved performance. Having a strong "core" (abdominals and lower back) will make most physical things you do much easier. Your middle section is where much of your power flows through. It's why most top golfers, swimmers, tennis players, and runners "play from the hips." Having good, strong abs will also relieve back pain, since most back pain comes from weak abdominals and tight back muscles.

How do you create strong abdominals? All you really need are ten crunches held for ten seconds three times a week. That's it. To perform the perfect crunch, lie with your back flat on the floor and your legs bent with feet flat on the ground shoulder width apart. With your hands behind your head, raise your head up just six inches—using your abs, not your arms—and hold a tight crunch for ten seconds. Really visualize all of your abs working.

Now how do you begin to see—and show off—your new abs? Ready? You already have them. *Everyone* has a decent set of abs. Your milkman, your neighbor, and, yes, you. If you want to *see* those great abs, the trick is not working your stomach constantly, it is liberating your abs from the shield of blubber around them. For that, focus more on long, sustained, fat-burning aerobic exercise (tip #67), not crunches or Abdo-Blaster machines. Spot reducing is a myth. Bottom line: Aerobic exercise burns fat, and fat is hiding your wonderful abdominals.

~~~~~~

ACTION ITEM

For the next month, do ten crunches three times a week. Combine that with smarter, fat-burning exercise and you will have strong, great-looking abs after just thirty days. And it won't cost you a penny.

67. Stay Aerobic

~~~~~~

Exercising at too high an intensity is one of the most detrimental errors people make in their fitness routines. Here's the secret to long-term fitness progress and performance: You don't ever need to work out to the point at which you are out of breath. This will come as a shock to most people who exercise under the "harder is better" ethic.

Let's quickly distinguish between anaerobic and aerobic exercise. As we learned in tip #23, your anaerobic threshold is the only number you need to know when exercising. When you work out aerobically, your body has plenty of oxygen present and uses fat as its primary fuel source. During exercise, your body feels good, you feel happy. You finish the workout feeling invigorated. As you increase the intensity and run low on oxygen, your body goes "anaerobic" and shifts to using sugar as fuel. Your body feels tight and your lungs burn. You finish the workout feeling exhausted.

If you work out at a comfortably challenging pace, you will become *fit without fatigue*—building energy over time rather than wearing yourself out. You will get injured less, and your workouts will stay fresh. This will lead to more passion and performance than any amount of anaerobic exercise. This is not to say you shouldn't challenge yourself. You should push into that "upper aerobic" area at least once a week, but even at that level, you are still "within yourself," and your breath rate, although deep and strong, is not out of control.

During your breakthrough sessions (tip #60), you should move into that anaerobic zone. The point here is that your workouts should be aerobic 95 percent of the time.

This applies to you serious athletes out there as well. Mark Allen, the greatest triathlete ever, was very strict about training aerobically. He likened aerobic exercise to building an engine and anaerobic exercise to turbocharging that engine. I like Allen's observation that most people are "trying to turbocharge one-cylinder engines." Your aerobic workouts will build a bigger, stronger aerobic engine. Allen would exercise relentlessly at 150 heartbeats per minute. Over the months, Allen would get faster and stronger at those lower heart rates. In January, he might cycle at twenty-one miles an hour at 150 beats per minute. In March, Allen would hum along at twenty-three miles per hour at the same comfortable heart rate. By race season, Allen's aerobic engine would power him along at an astounding twenty-eight miles an hour. His effort would remain under control while his competition would suffer at astronomical heart rates. Allen was an "aerobic juggernaut" because he had the patience and vision to build his aerobic engine.

ACTION ITEM

Pay close attention to your heart rates, and breath rates, during exercise. Keep the majority of your workouts aerobic. Exercising this way takes enormous patience, but after just two weeks, you will feel stronger, healthier, and fitter.

68. Consult the Experts

Do not consider it proof just because it is written in books, for a liar who will deceive with his tongue will not hesitate to do the same with his pen.

—MAIMONIDES, PHILOSOPHER (1135–1204)

This tip could save you more time and money than any other in this book. There are a lot of people out there telling you a lot of different things about fitness and nutrition. Many of these people simply do not know as much as they claim they do; and a few will tell you anything you want to hear just to sell you something, particularly in today's fitness industry.

To achieve your fitness goals, you must consult the real experts. When you speak with a bona fide expert about something important to you, you can learn more in one hour than you might through trial and error in one year. When I began my triathlon career, I thought I knew it all. I'd routinely ignore the wisdom of the older guys, because I was too preoccupied with climbing the triathlon mountain as quickly as possible. Instead, however, I spent the first two years running around the base of that mountain, wasting lots of energy. At last I gave in and decided my energy would be better channeled if I consulted the real experts. I asked myself, Who is the most successful person in my sport right now? At the time, it was Mark Allen. So while in Finland, I sat with Mark and asked him for his sage counsel.

Allen's advice: "Don't overrace, train aerobically, and be patient in your training, your racing, and your life." I took those words very seriously, since that was sixteen years of wisdom condensed into thirty seconds. Those simple words changed my career.

ACTION ITEM

Assess your fitness and decide what needs to be dealt with by an expert—it could be an injury or an annoying plateau in your fitness. Solicit the advice of a high-level expert who has been there, someone you trust unequivocally. This will be some of the most valuable time you've ever spent on your fitness.

69. Don't Buy In to the Supplement Hype

If exercise could be packed in a pill, it would be the single most widely prescribed and beneficial medicine in the nation.

—NATIONAL INSTITUTE ON AGING

A question I am often asked is *Which nutritional supplements are hype, which ones work, and how do I use those to see and feel results now, so that by summer I can have a butt roughly one-third the size of my current butt?* My response: "Ninety-nine percent of nutritional supplements do not work. And the 1 percent that do work do not come close to the effects of simple exercise."

The nutritional supplement industry has become a four-ring circus: hundreds of companies bombard us with countless products, exaggerated ads, and sleazy marketing tactics. The result? Too many products, too much misinformation, and nobody to trust. These days, people are seeking to "pay" for their fitness more than ever before, when all the answers are found in simple exercise and intelligent eating.

In my personal pursuit to gain a competitive advantage, I've experimented with just about every legal nutritional supplement there is, and I've come to this firm belief: Virtually all nutritional supplements are not nearly worth the money.

The only supplements you need that are proven to work in the real world are antioxidants (vitamins A, C, E, zinc, and selenium). A powerful multivitamin twice a day will help to prevent illness, offset the free-radical damage from exercise, and keep your energy levels up. There is no significant difference between most brands of supplements. In fact, I use generic supplements and they work as well on my body as any name brand I've used. Not having to deal with the guesswork and expense of buying all sorts of nutritional supplements ought to save you a good deal of time and money.

ACTION ITEM
Take antioxidants day and night. When you're tempted to purchase nutritional supplements beyond that, turn your attention instead to exercise and go for a nice one-hour hike. That hike will provide ten times the benefit of any supplement you can buy.

70. Sex Is Where Passion and Exercise Intersect

The idea here is that in terms of aerobic fitness, heartbeats are heartbeats. If your heart is humming along in your aerobic zone (tip #23), you are reaping optimal cardiovascular benefits. So whether you are running on a treadmill, swimming in a lake, playing tennis, or having passionate sex, you are boosting your fitness level. The activity you choose is entirely up to you.

Now is the time to break free from the idea of suffering through physical activities you dislike simply because you think it's the only path to better fitness. Contrary to conventional wisdom, running on a treadmill is not going to make you fitter than dancing, playing a hearty game of tennis, or power-hiking up a mountainside with a loved one. Heartbeats are heartbeats.

ACTION ITEM

Constantly vary your physical activities and be creative with finding new ways to stay fit. Always strive to keep your exercise fun, fresh, and passion-driven. I cannot think of another activity that is more passion-driven and better for your heart than sex!

71. Go Longer, Less Frequently

This tip is about how best to allocate your time to get the most benefit from aerobic exercise.

The traditional advice for aerobic exercise is "Twenty minutes, three times a week." Unfortunately, that ain't nearly gonna cut it. To reap the real aerobic or fat-burning effects from exercise, you've got to work out for at least forty-five minutes at a time. It is much more beneficial to do three 45-minute sessions per week than five 20-minute workouts. Here's why:

Your aerobic system takes a while to get rolling along. It's a delicate process: you must eat low-glycemic foods beforehand to minimize insulin production (tip #57), your warm-up needs to be gradual (tip #14), and you need to monitor your intensity level during exercise (tip #23). If you can get your aerobic system churning along, you will realize enormous benefits in health, body fat management, and athletic performance.

Only *after* twenty minutes of continuous aerobic exercise does your body begin to absorb the benefits of aerobic exercise. It is only then that you begin burning body fat (about a gram a minute). After twenty minutes, your cardio-vascular system is in full swing and the endorphins begin to flow.

~~~~~~

ACTION ITEM

Modify your program to include longer aerobic sessions—even if it means you must cut back on frequency, it is well worth the trade-off.

72. Everything You Need to Know About Nutrition Boils Down to Twelve Words

Food is an important part of a balanced diet.
—FRAN LEBOWITZ, WRITER

It's evident that in order to rise above the clamor, today's nutrition authors must develop supercatchy titles and design bright, bold packaging—or their books will not sell. Books like *Blood Type Diet, Caveman Diet,* and *The Peanut Butter Diet* (my favorite) crowd the shelves of bookstores. But are these books really helping? I don't think so.

We are awash in more nutrition and diet information than ever, and as a nation, we are fatter than we've ever been. Many of today's nutrition books spend hundreds of pages telling you what they could in one sentence. People are fed up.

Here's all you need to know about a high-performance diet for the rest of your life: *Graze on visually balanced, low-glycemic foods your body wants.*

➤ **"Graze . . ."** Throw out the three squares a day and eat smaller portions throughout the day. When you eat more than six hundred calories at one sitting, your body stores the rest as body fat. Since blood sugar levels determine your energy levels, you should graze every few hours on two-hundred-to-three-hundred-calorie low-sugar, protein-oriented snacks (bagel with low-fat cream cheese, turkey sandwich, yogurt, and so on). Your energy will grow, and your waistline will shrink. Eating five to six small meals during the day helps us avoid overeating after eight P.M.

➤ **". . . on visually balanced . . ."** Your eyes can tell you everything you need to know about the ideal macronutrient composition of your meals. When you sit down to eat, just have a look at your food and ask this question: *Does this meal have reasonable proportions of protein, carbohydrates, and quality fats, in the right amounts?* It's really as simple as that.

➤ **". . . low-glycemic foods . . ."** The most important thing you need to know about choosing foods is where they appear on the glycemic index (appendix B). The glycemic index is a scale that rates how quickly food elevates your blood sugar. To keep your insulin down and your energy constant, eat more low-glycemic foods throughout the day. After workouts, however, aim for foods higher up on the index: sweets, carbos, and so on (tip #57).

➤ **". . . your body wants."** This is the most important part of the sentence. Over time, we've been taught to abdicate our knowledge of nutrition to these authors. Yet if I had to choose who knew more about your nutrition, a world-renowned nutritionist or you, I'd choose you. Without a doubt. You are the best coach for your body, not some doctor or nutritionist! You have all the answers about optimum nutrition inside of you; it's literally woven into your genetic code. As you develop a deeper body awareness, you will be able to make all of your own food decisions as opposed to looking to others for those answers. After you learn to hear your body's signals, if it asks for Ben & Jerry's once in a while, dig in. Your body will thank you.

73. Use Relaxed Strength

~~~~~~

The less effort, the faster and more powerful you will be.
—BRUCE LEE, MARTIAL ARTS EXPERT, ACTOR (1940–1973)

Have you ever felt a baby's grip? How can they clamp on to your nose with such astonishing strength without any developed muscles? It is because babies are the most natural athletes in the world. They are using "relaxed strength"—an advanced performance concept at the highest levels of athletic competition. If you learn to apply this technique to your fitness, no matter what your fitness level, you will perform at a higher level and enjoy workouts more.

Right now, get down on the floor and do a push-up with every muscle in your body fully tensed. Do it slowly, and *try* as hard as you can. Take ten seconds to rest. Now do another push-up, this time without "trying." Just relax, and glide up effortlessly while exhaling as if someone is pulling you up from the floor.

You've just experienced the difference between how a novice and a top-level athlete perform exercise. Top athletes' minds are as calm and relaxed as the eye, and their bodies are as dynamic as the hurricane. Be as effortless as possible in your next workout. Keep your effort up, but your body relaxed. Do this and you will be functioning at a world-class level regardless of your performance.

74. Approach How You Eat with More Reverence

We need to reestablish a positive relationship with food, so I'm not going to tell you what to eat. You've got enough people telling you that. This is much simpler; it's about *how* to eat.

One interesting common trait among the very best athletes with whom I have trained, the Olympic champions, is that they give exceptional reverence to how and when they eat. It's not a matter of what they eat—I've seen these people down burgers and fries, pizza, and candy bars! Hey, you've got to be bad sometimes, right? If you focus more on how you eat, your nutritional health will improve from the inside out. Here are some suggestions:

➤ Make more simple, healthy, home-cooked meals for yourself. The act of preparing your food encourages you to treat meals with more reverence.

➤ Eating in front of the television is an instant disconnect between you and your food. We've all overeaten while watching television at some point. Best to eat before or after television.

➤ Set the mood. A comfortable environment while eating will relax your mood and improve your digestion.

➤ Chew well: the digestive process begins with chewing. You will extract more nutritional value from food if you eat more slowly. In addition, it takes about twenty minutes for the "fullness response" to kick in, so by chewing more slowly, you will more likely eat the right amount of food.

➤ Experience the totality of food. Eating should be a complete experience: the anticipation, the preparation, the presentation, the aromas, the tastes, and the satisfaction after eating a good meal. As you begin to appreciate food on a deeper level, you will be inspired to treat it with more reverence.

75. Focus More on Quality Proteins

By now, you've been inundated with books and advice compelling you to eat more protein and fewer carbohydrates. It's true. Americans have never been fatter and have never eaten less fat! It's not so much the dietary fat that's making us fat, it is the overconsumption of sugar and carbohydrates. There is no doubt that if you eat less bread and pasta, you will lose body fat. But you don't need an entire book to tell you that: just focus more on quality proteins.

We overconsume carbohydrates because they are simply more convenient to eat: bagels, cereals, and so on. I'm as susceptible to this as anyone; in fact, I've been known to eat eleven energy bars in one day, simply because they are so quick and easy to eat. I can't say I felt like a million bucks at the end of the day, however.

Eat at least one lean, quality protein per day: fish, egg whites, lean ground beef, tofu, or beans. If you do that while avoiding the "simple" carbohydrates like white flour and sugar, your waistline will shrink and your energy will grow.

76. Let Your Body's Instincts Have the Final Word

'I've been giving you a lot of specific advice in this book, but you must be open to modifying that advice to fit your body and your lifestyle. You know your body better than anyone. Today there are more people telling you what to do with your exercise and nutrition than ever before. It's overbearing, expensive, and confusing. It's almost as if the fitness industry is trying to convince us that we're the *last* people we can trust.

The best athletes in the world turn inside for their answers. I suggest you do the same. You have enough instincts to know when, how, and what to eat. As you develop your body awareness, you will even understand exactly when and how you should exercise.

For the first ten minutes of every workout, "listen" to the signals your body is sending. Your body will literally guide you through the entire workout: how much, how hard, how long. (One caveat: Unless you are sick or injured, don't listen to your mind *before* workouts. It will give you every reason not to get out there. I've invariably had my best workouts when I was convinced I couldn't get off the couch.) It's important to learn as much as you can about fitness, but trust your instincts. This empowering self-reliance will become far more reliable and valuable to you than any video, book, or fad.

77. Scrutinize Food Labels Before You Buy

This is not a conspiracy theory, but doesn't it seem as though food manufacturers are trying to hide things from us? They used to freely print "sugar" on the list of ingredients in foods, until we all learned sugar was driving our insulin skyward and our bellies outward. If you look at food labels today, sugar has been changed to "evaporated cane juice." *Evaporated cane juice.*

Here are a few ways to ensure that you make the best food choices while at the grocery store:

➤ "Fat-free" rarely means sugar-free, and it definitely doesn't mean calorie-free. You can eat a completely fat-free diet and still be overweight. Don't buy something simply because it's "fat-free." Pay more attention to the nutritional value and the sugar content.

➤ Generally, the fewer the ingredients the better. If reading the list of ingredients of a certain food requires more than five minutes and a magnifying glass, something is wrong. Go for foods that are made simply.

➤ Watch for "partially hydrogenated oils." These types of oils are very detrimental to your health. You'll find hydrogenated oils in cookies, crackers, and chips.

➤ Other terms for sugar are (in order from best to worst) fructose, honey, molasses, sucrose, glucose, and, yes, evaporated cane juice.

78. Be Satisfied with the Here and Now

It's human nature to want more, particularly when it relates to our bodies. We want bigger muscles, smaller waistlines, and tighter abs. I've met very few people who are truly happy with their bodies or level of fitness, and that includes the best athletes in the world.

As a nation, we stand out in our obsessive compulsion with looking thin. America's irrational focus on body fat makes it virtually impossible for us to enjoy how we look. It's time to disengage yourself from that craziness. First you need to realize that comparing yourself to supermodels or professional athletes does little for your self-esteem. If you must measure yourself against others, use everyday people.

Next, accept that life is here and it is now. It doesn't begin when you are 9 percent body fat. This strategy is not about relaxing your standards—you should be demanding more from your body, not accepting less. However, having high standards does not require that you be hard on yourself. This is about being happy with where you are *right now*.

~~~~~~

During workouts, celebrate your body. Revel in your ability to exercise, because I can assure you, this marvelous privilege could be revoked at any moment. Think broadly about how fortunate you are to be able to exercise. In the grand scheme of things, moving your body at will is an exceptional thing to be able to do. The purpose of your workouts should be to build your confidence and your passion more than making you thin or fast. If you focus on the here and now, the destination of a fitter you will come and the journey will have been enjoyed.

79. Create a World-Class Shopping List

To lose weight and boost your energy levels, you don't need to spend a *penny* on weight loss fads, exercise machines, pills, potions, or lotions. Simply create your own "world-class shopping list" and stick to it; that way the bad stuff doesn't make it home. Here are the ten best foods taken from the grocery lists of some of the world's best athletes; you may want to add some of these foods to your cart the next time around:

➤ **Tomatoes.** These are a good source of the powerful antioxidant *lycopene*, which has been shown to reduce the risk of cancer by 35 percent. Concentrated tomato sauces (fresh pizza and pasta sauces) contain much more lycopene than fresh tomatoes.

➤ **Extra-virgin olive oil (and all "healthy fats").** "Good fats" balance your hormonal system, satisfy your appetite, and boost your immunity. In addition, many widely respected nutritionists claim that olive oil is the main dietary reason for low mortality rates among Mediterranean populations. Opt for extra-virgin, cold-pressed olive oil. It is well worth the nominal extra expense.

➤ **Red grapes.** This fruit is loaded with health-producing phytonutrients and antioxidants—and yes, it's true: moderate consumption of red wine increases health and longevity.

➤ **Nuts.** Recent Harvard research found that eating five ounces of nuts a week can cut heart attack deaths by 40 percent. Nuts are high in fat, but most are the good type: monounsaturated and/or omega-3. Peanuts, walnuts, and almonds are the best.

➤ **Whole grains.** A new University of Minnesota study suggests that the more whole grains you eat, the lower your odds of death. Whole grains contain anticancer agents and help stabilize blood sugar and insulin levels, which is vital for health and fitness.

➤ **Salmon (and other fatty fish).** Contains high amounts of the type of fat, omega-3, that performs miracles throughout the body, fighting virtually every chronic disease known. Just be sure your fish is as fresh as possible, and aim for two servings a week.

- **Blueberries.** One of the highest foods in antioxidants. Powerful antiaging properties . . . and just so darn delicious!
- **Garlic.** Arguably the most powerful disease and ailment fighter on the planet.
- **Spinach.** Spinach is second among vegetables only to garlic in antioxidant activity. It's also rich in folic acid, which helps prevent heart disease, cancer, and mental disorders. Avoid cooking spinach, or any vegetables, too long, as this reduces the nutritional content.
- **Tea.** One cup of green or black tea per day cuts heart disease risk in half. If you have a choice between black and green, you know how I feel about green (tip #51).

ACTION ITEM

Tear out appendix C and bring that with you to the grocery store. You don't need to stick exclusively to that list, just add a few of those foods to your shopping cart each time you shop and your nutritional health will improve.

80. Pay More Attention to Water

If you apply one health-related tip from this book, make it this one. Dehydration is a serious health problem in America. A recent study in the *Journal of American Medicine* showed that a whopping 83 percent of Americans are "chronically dehydrated." Our bodies are 75 percent water, yet we consume, on average, just forty ounces of water a day. Those are pretty scary numbers.

Dehydration's real danger lies in its insidiousness. Often you cannot feel it directly, but dehydration manifests itself in headaches, fatigue, irritability, and illness. When my body isn't feeling right, the first thing I do is drink a few glasses of water, which most often cures my ills. The world's best athletes carry water with them wherever they go. You should, too.

If you drink more water, you will get more benefit from your exercise, your skin will look healthier, your physical activity will feel easier, you will recover more quickly, you will burn more fat during exercise, and your energy levels and immunity will improve. I'd say that's worth the ten glasses a day you need to drink.

However, it's not enough to drink more water; the water needs to be clean. There are over 450,000 unregulated dumps in this country, and that pollutes much of our water supply. In addition, there are no regulations on bottled "spring water"—that water could be running out of the tap of some guy named Roy in Arkansas. *Distilled* water is the only kind that is guaranteed clean. Michael Colgan, one of the world's leading nutritionists, insists that in order to reach your fitness potential, you must drink distilled water. From my personal experience, I agree.

~~~~~~

ACTION ITEM

Begin your day right by drinking two tall glasses of water upon arising. Keep water close to you all day, every day: one water bottle on your desk at work and one in your car. Just having water near you will remind you to drink it. If you drink more clean water, you will realize powerful gains in your health.

81. Fast

~~~~~~

Not eating may seem like an extreme or esoteric thing to do, but it can boost your health and fitness on several different levels.

Most of us tend to eat more food than our bodies need. We are constantly processing that food, which requires a lot of energy from our bodies and is one reason you feel tired after big meals. Overeating also contributes to various diseases. Short-term fasting is a safe, proven therapy that will boost your health. Here are some things that a fast will do for you:

➤ Fasting will thoroughly cleanse years of toxins stored in your body. During a fast, your body metabolizes fat where some toxins have been stored for years.

➤ When you come off the fast, you will be more sensitive to what and how you eat. This is an enormously important skill to develop, since it is the most surefire way to make the right food choices for the rest of your life.

➤ After some initial feelings of hunger (twenty-four hours), you will experience periods of profound mental clarity, in part because your energies are directed to your brain, not your belly.

➤ Your body will be freed up to heal itself more efficiently. Because digestion takes such a large amount of energy, your body has to put the healing of other tissues on hold. During a fast, your body can turn more of its attention to healing your body.

ACTION ITEM

Begin a two-day fast sometime over the next thirty days. You may want to fast over a weekend, since fasting may make you tired. During your fast, drink plenty of water. You may want to accelerate the detoxification process by taking hot baths, getting some sunlight, and napping often. You may even want to get a deep-tissue massage to really unlock those deeply stored toxins. If you truly tune in to your body, by the end of your fast you will feel like a different person. That much I can assure you.

82. During Workouts, Look Inside

I believe that the best medium for self-improvement is not when you're sitting in a seminar, it's when you are in dynamic motion. Have you ever noticed how a good, long exercise session can instantly bring clarity to tough life issues? Exercise has a way of stripping away our veneers. The primitive, pure act of exercise seems to bring out deep issues we tend to avoid in daily life.

This is not to say self-improvement seminars don't help. They do. The point is that in exercise you can resolve a lot of personal issues *while you improve your body.* And the passion generated from improving your body will be more permanent than that gained at a self-help seminar or from an inspiring book. If you're a big believer in seminars, then take what you learn in the classroom and let those lessons sink in while you exercise. You may even want to listen to motivational tapes while you work out.

~~~~~~

ACTION ITEM

During one workout this week, take an objective look at your life: where you are and where you're headed. I have come to the most important life decisions during periods of exceptional mental clarity brought on by exercise. I hope you do as well.

83. When Your Athletic Shoes Wear Out, Give Them to a Homeless Shelter

Serious runners discard their running shoes after three hundred to four hundred miles. That's smart: wearing running shoes for too long increases the risk of injury. But what you do with those shoes after you're done can make all the difference. If every runner in this country donated their used running shoes to homeless shelters, every homeless person would have a few pairs of perfectly good shoes!

Last year I donated two hundred pairs of sponsored shoes to a homeless shelter in my hometown. That week, almost every homeless person I saw had a bright white pair of running shoes standing in stark contrast with their dark clothing. It warmed my heart as much as anything I've ever done.

When your shoes—or any athletic gear, for that matter—become too worn for you, donate them to a homeless shelter. Better yet, start a drive for athletic gear in your hometown and call the entire community to action.

84. When You Lace Up the Shoes, Tone Down the Ego

~~~~~~

This one is more for the men out there. Guys, we've got to chill out. Our egos get us into all sorts of trouble, and they block the way to increased athletic performance and greater enjoyment of life. Plus, we infuriate the women out there with our overbearing egos.

It's ironic that early in my career, when I had everything to prove, I trained fueled almost exclusively by my ego. I would "race" everyone I saw out on the roads. As I became more successful in my sport, that ego was replaced with a calm, quiet confidence. I stuck to my program and listened to my body during workouts, and my athletic performance shot through the roof.

This is not about confidence. Confidence is a must. Ego is a different creature. It tricks us into doing things that can be totally detrimental to our fitness—like going massively anaerobic just to demoralize a total stranger who cycles past us on an easy Sunday bike ride. In fitness, you'll perform much better if you let go of your ego. Let that weekend warrior whiz by you if you're on a rest day. That's how the pros do it.

The irony is, the more ego you display, the more obvious it is to everyone that secretly you're afraid you're a dork. There will always be people who are better than you at your sport. It's okay to be competitive, just lay off the macho thing. Your body will thank you. The women out there will thank you as well.

85. There Are 168 Hours in the Week— Give at Least Four of Them to Your Body

This tip is about prioritizing. There is one certainty in life: We live in this body until we die. We have a choice to live in a body that helps us reach our potential or one that limits us. When we develop a higher-performance body, we absolutely begin to live with more passion. We must commit to giving more time to our fitness right here, right now.

Unfortunately, people's busy lives push their fitness to the back burner, and over time they accept a body that functions at half steam. And they don't realize it. They forget what it feels like to have limitless energy. Although we are all busy, there is plenty of time to get it all in. If fitting in at least four hours a week requires some changes in your life, then you must do that.

There are 168 hours in a week. You spend 50 working, 50 sleeping and resting. That leaves you with 68 to do the rest. This month, give at least 4 hours each week to your fitness.

86. Laugh More During Exercise

So you laugh out loud during exercise? Why not? Oh, right, your fitness is serious business. But it should also be fun. There is no question that when your workouts become more fun, they will feel easier and you will perform better. Physiologically, when you laugh, your body releases healthy chemicals, your blood pressure comes down, and your muscles relax.

I've found the best way to include laughter during workouts is to train with others. Every Saturday I ride with a group of people who make me laugh hysterically. These are, by far, my most productive and enjoyable workouts. Four hours can fly by, and I will not have given one thought to the pain or duration of the workout. These guys keep me in such good spirits that the workout is over before I know it. The best part is, I cannot wait for the next group ride. This sort of excitement and passion about workouts will take your physical and mental performance to another level.

ACTION ITEM

Approach your workouts with a new level of humor. The best way to do this is to work out with bigger groups of people once or twice a week. Within that group, find people with whom you really connect, people who make you laugh. Begin to schedule one or two sessions with that smaller group each week. This is one of the most important things you can do for your passion and performance in fitness.

87. Running Gives You the Most Fat-Burning Bang for Your Workout Buck

For cardiovascular fitness and fat burning, running is king. Just look at the world's top marathon runners. They have zero body fat. Running is a high-intensity, weight-bearing activity. Since there is nothing "supporting" you—a bicycle or water, for example—your body's natural tendency is to get as light as possible. If you weigh 170 pounds, every time you land while running, your body absorbs up to 800 pounds of pressure per square inch. Your body adapts to that direct high impact by lightening the load. In addition, running is a continuous aerobic activity, which burns the most body fat (tip #67).

One problem with running, however, is that it carries a high risk of injury. Here are a few suggestions that will reduce your risk of running-induced injury:

- No matter what your level, do not run more than five days a week. If you do, you're just asking for trouble.
- Hit the weight room and develop balanced strength. Many running injuries come not from muscular weakness, but from muscular *imbalance*. To develop balanced strength, isolate your muscles with single-arm and single-leg exercises. Dumbbells work best.
- Stretch after workouts. Muscles that tighten up from running are your feet, calves, hamstrings, and low back. It's important to stretch easily after workouts, while your muscles are warm.
- Head to your nearest running specialty store and ask the experts to determine which shoes best suit *your individual biomechanics*. There are countless types of running shoes, and today's technology can dramatically improve your running experience. Running shoes are not the place to save money.
- Run on soft, even surfaces. Wide, well-surfaced trails are best. Concrete sidewalks are the worst.
- Refine your technique. Subtle errors in technique, like overstriding, can lead to chronic injuries. Run with an experienced runner and learn from him or her.

If you can reduce the risk of injury, running will provide you with tremendous cardiovascular and fat-burning benefits in addition to a new mental and spiritual freedom.

88. Get Bodywork at Least Once a Month

etting some form of bodywork—massage, chiropractic, or acupuncture—is one of the most important things you can do for your physical and spiritual health. Bodywork can be costly, but you deserve it!

A deep-tissue massage will not only relax you mentally, it will eliminate harmful toxins from your body. Most people feel that bodywork is a luxury, but once you get it, you wonder how you did without it. Top athletes view bodywork as essential "tune-ups" that keep their bodies running smoothly and, more important, keep them from getting injured. Bodywork is preventative medicine that can dramatically improve your overall wellness.

ACTION ITEM This month, get a one-hour bodywork session. This can be chiropractic, deep-tissue massage, even acupuncture. Finding someone who really knows bodywork can make the difference between a fair and a *stunning* experience. Here are two additional suggestions: The trick is to relax more on days you get body-work—if you let yourself stress out that same day, you've just wasted $60. To make bodywork more affordable, solicit local bodyworker schools. The students at these schools need a certain number of hours to fulfill their degree requirements, so the prices are lower than those of certified bodyworkers. These student bodyworkers are just as good as any you'll find because they're focused on doing a *textbook* job.

89. Exercise with a Dog

~~~~~~

Animals create vibrant health in people. A dog's passion for life is infectious; they lift our spirits and keep us present in the moment. None of the athletes with whom I have trained can match the unbridled passion of my Bernese mountain dog, Ally.

Animals have an enviable present-moment awareness and love of physical activity. Have you ever watched a dog play at the beach? I just love watching this awesome display of "exercise passion." Dogs get wild with excitement at beaches: sprinting across the sand, writhing wildly on their backs, and, without reason, barking at the ocean. Sometimes, when I get myopic in my training, when I totally forget why I am a professional triathlete, I go to the beach with Ally and watch her play for hours. That invariably puts a smile on my face and reminds me that the *sheer act of movement* is, in itself, a passion-driven activity. It just reminds me that we're so damn lucky to be alive.

Get out there with your dog. Play Frisbee. Run on the beach. Watch your dog closely during these moments—they are purely focused on the thrill of movement. If you don't own a dog, take a "shelter" dog with you. They could use the time outside just as much as you could use the exercise.

90. The Five Best Fat-Burning Secrets

I predict that the two most read strategies in this book will be "Be Bad" (tip #15) and this one. It seems everyone loves to burn more body fat, even athletes—who know that using fat as fuel is more efficient than using sugar.

Losing weight is one the most confusing, frustrating, annoying, costly, and exhausting battles we face. Whether you are a couch potato at war with your love handles or a three-day-a-week cyclist trying to ride off those last five pounds, losing weight is a nagging problem. The proliferation of weight loss pills, potions, fads, and contraptions don't seem to help us much, either.

I believe that real fitness is a matter of how you feel more than how you look. However, my fiancée said if I didn't include this strategy on burning body fat, she'd "kickbox me on behalf of all women." So, without further ado, here are five of the best ways to burn more body fat during exercise:

➤ **Drink caffeinated green tea.** Caffeine is a powerful workout supplement that has been shown to increase the amount of fat burned during aerobic exercise. Caffeine mobilizes free fatty acids in the bloodstream, but it takes about an hour before that happens. Drink one to two cups of green tea forty-five to sixty minutes before a workout. Since your body "builds up resistance to" the effects of caffeine over time, try to reserve your green tea for bigger workouts.

➤ **Stay aerobic.** To use fat as fuel during exercise, your body must have plenty of oxygen present, so for maximum fat loss, do not exercise to the point where you're gasping for air (tip #67). When it needs oxygen, your body has no choice but to switch its fuel source from body fat to sugar. The best way to ensure you're exercising in the "fat-burning zone" is to wear a heart rate monitor during exercise.

➤ **Run.** You get the most fat-burning bang for your buck by jogging at a moderate, aerobic pace (tip #87). Period.

➤ **Train for an athletic event.** This may be the most effective strategy, because when you are exercising with a specific goal in mind, you focus more on the excitement of training for that event than on the fat-burning part.

Ironically, you will burn a lot more fat that way, because you are training more consistently and with more passion.

➤ **Exercise on an empty stomach.** This isn't the most exciting prospect, but there is no doubt that when you exercise without eating beforehand, your body uses more body fat as fuel. This is particularly true of exercising first thing in the morning. In fact, some researchers have found that twenty minutes of exercise first thing in the morning on an empty stomach will burn more fat than a one-hour session later in the day after eating food. It's best to have some protein and fat about an hour before your workout, but if fast weight loss is your singular goal, exercising on an empty stomach is most effective.

Putting all of these tips together is how some of the world's best athletes "strip down" before major athletic competitions. They wake up, drink two cups of strong coffee, wait forty-five minutes, strap on a heart rate monitor, then run for an hour or more, without eating anything beforehand. This isn't exactly the *healthiest* way to lose body fat, but I have lost up to six pounds of pure body fat in a week using this technique.

91. Be Selfish About Your Fitness

Most people—bosses, usually—would rather see you working than exercising. Unless we have a strong dedication to our fitness, or an encouraging group of workout buddies around us (tip #28), we get very little social support for maintaining our fitness.

Some of us may view being selfish about our fitness as vanity. Wrong. Improving our bodies will improve our self-esteem and our interpersonal relationships. Our passion for fitness will rub off on the people around us.

ACTION ITEM

From now on, your fitness needs to come first. This is your *body* we're talking about. Don't let others take the time you have reserved for your workouts.

Now that you've written your workouts into your daily planner (tip #41), you can politely decline those who want you to do something else. When you become a fitter, more alive human being, you become more valuable to those around you anyway.

92. Develop Simple, Positive Habits to Realize Profound Lifestyle Improvement

Many of the world's best athletes are not exceptionally gifted genetically; they just have stunningly good daily habits. They do powerful little things each day, and over time, the effects of those habits build them into champions.

There is no doubt that we are a product of our collective habits. For example, if you wake up and head straight to your computer every morning, the effects of that small habit will shape your fitness destiny. Subtle changes in habit are easy to make yet have potentially huge benefits. What would happen if, every morning, the first thing you did was run for forty-five minutes? My bet is that your life would change dramatically for the better.

Pull back and take note of your habits for two days. This is a wonderfully revealing exercise, because it gives you a new perspective on how you live day to day. In particular, watch what habits shape your health and fitness. Do you skip workouts for a similar reason every time? Are you especially skilled at talking yourself out of exercise (tip #39)? Becoming aware of your habits is the first step to replacing them with powerful, positive ones.

93. Real Fitness Is Less About How You Look, More About How You Feel

As a nation, America stands out in its obsessive compulsion with looking thin. Society's focus on body fat makes it virtually impossible for us to enjoy how we look. It is far better to have a stronger heart, stronger lungs, and a stronger sense of self-esteem than it is to be thin.

As you know, the skinny supermodels you see in the magazines are paid large amounts of money to look that way, but many of these people are not healthy. However, things are changing. For the first time since the sixties, people, particularly young people, are beginning to accept their bodies as they are.

Skinny is not healthy. Healthy is healthy. Early in my career, I believed that stripping my body of every ounce of body fat would lead to better athletic performances. I was relentless in my quest to forge my body into a piece of iron. As I got down to 5 percent, 4 percent, 3 percent body fat, my body was in turmoil. I was on the verge of illness, I had no energy, and I certainly did not enjoy my exercise. After two miserable performances at events, my fiancée convinced me to pack on some weight and enjoy myself. I did exactly that. And I won my next race by seven minutes.

~~~~~~

ACTION ITEM

Ditch the scale and all of the thoughts and beliefs attached to it. Number one, the scale shows you very little: muscle weighs more than fat, so the scale isn't telling you the right story anyway. Look at yourself in the mirror and decide if you are making progress. Number two: Constantly watching the scale is an emotional roller coaster. Begin to judge your fitness on how energetic, positive, and passionate you feel. That will redefine how you view your body, and you will begin to set things in motion that make you feel more energetic, positive, and passionate.

94. Work Out with Kids

The pursuit of truth and beauty is a sphere of activity in which we are permitted to remain children all our lives.

—ALBERT EINSTEIN, PHYSICIST (1879–1955)

Passion is as fleeting as it is powerful. It takes time and patience for the passion for exercise to become part of your soul. Periodically you've got to reignite that passion when it flames out, and one of the best ways I've found to do that is to exercise with kids. Children are masters of passion, and they can be powerful teachers if you listen with an open heart and a clear mind. In fact, most top athletes I know have a childlike passion for their sport, and it is one reason they can perform such dazzling athletic feats.

ACTION ITEM

Play your favorite sport with a child. Enjoy this time, fully letting your mind go. Be present in the moment. Carry this new childlike passion for your sport back to your regular workouts. When your exercise becomes boring, draw upon the lessons you learned from your time with those masters of passion.

95. Your First Thoughts and Actions Set the Tone for the Day—Make Them Good Ones

Sometimes the day gets away from us and we don't find time for our health or fitness. Most top athletes start the morning with "rituals" that prepare their bodies and minds for optimal functioning all day.

The mornings provide an ideal time to boost your physical health while taking a moment to mentally prepare a strong, enduring inner peace, all of which will lead to a more enjoyable and productive day. My personal morning routine consists of water, breathing, sunlight, and "mental centering." Right when I wake up, I drink a tall glass of water, do a few deep belly breaths, and clear my mind of all negative feelings. Three minutes and I feel mentally and physically ready for a world-class day.

ACTION ITEM

Develop your own simple morning ritual. It doesn't need to be complex. In fact, it can be as short as thirty seconds. Just wake up with your morning routine and stick to it for two weeks. Your days may become much more productive from this one simple habit.

96. Exercise Based on Time, Not Distance

This may seem like a small point, but it's not. Training based on time is how most top professional endurance athletes exercise. Here's why:

Your body doesn't "understand" distance; it understands time. A seven-mile run in the mountains on a cold day is far more stressful to your system than a seven-mile run on a flat surface in sixty-five-degree weather.

Some of us get obsessed with fulfilling certain distances per workout or per week, and that can lead to overtraining. Exercising based on time will free you up from the constraints of having to cover specific distances, sometimes over awkward terrain. This will lead to more enjoyable workouts.

ACTION ITEM

For the next week, measure the duration of your exercise on time instead of distance. If you are a thirty-mile-per-week runner, become a five-hour-per-week runner. In cycling, go for "an hour" instead of "twenty miles." Don't concern yourself with the distance. Just start your watch, free your mind, and go.

97. Strength Training Is a Must (Particularly for Women)

Lifting weights will do as much to ensure your long-term physical well-being as anything you will ever do. You lose half a pound of muscle every year after age thirty, and this has drastic effects on your health and fitness.

Women have a special need for strength training since it is so effective at building bone density, which can prevent osteoporosis. One hour of strength work twice a week will improve posture, maintain muscle tissue, boost energy levels, increase bone density, prevent injury, and improve your resiliency. And muscle requires a lot of calories for maintenance: for every pound of muscle you add, you burn eight to twelve pounds of fat per year!

Commit to at least two 1-hour gym sessions a week. Any less, you won't improve. Any more, diminishing returns. Generally, all you need during each workout is two "sets" of seven exercises covering your entire body in this order: quadriceps, chest, hamstrings, back, calves, shoulders, abdominals. Rest for twenty to thirty seconds between each "set" and one minute between each exercise.

Using flawless technique will bring the fastest and most enduring results in the gym: exhale during the "lift" and inhale on the "recovery." Go through your full range of motion to improve flexibility. Focus on, and isolate, the specific muscle you're using. For example, don't throw your back into bench presses—that works your back, not your chest! If you want real results, you've got to work hard in the weight room.

Here are suggestions to achieve different personal objectives:

➤ To build muscle mass, lift fewer repetitions with heavier weight. Sets should be in the ten, six, four repetition range, lifting to "failure" in the last reps of each set.
➤ For overall muscle tone and strength, lift more repetitions (twenty, fifteen, twelve) at a lighter weight and move quickly from machine to machine. This will build aerobic strength concurrently with muscular strength.
➤ To build speed and stamina, lift the weight in an explosive fashion and re-

turn to the starting point more slowly. This will develop your fast-twitch muscle fibers and increase your muscular coordination.

One of the best ways to simplify your exercise program is to buy a few sets of dumbbells and lift at home. This saves you the monthly gym fees and the time and energy involved in preparing for gym workouts.

98. Blame Less and You'll Perform More

People are always blaming their circumstances for what they are. I don't believe in circumstances. The people who get on in this world are the people who get up and look for the circumstances they want and, if they can't find them, make them.

—GEORGE BERNARD SHAW, WRITER (1856–1950)

Blame disempowers you. Plain and simple. We waste enormous amounts of energy pointing the finger at others, when we should be looking inside and resolving the issues at hand. This is particularly true of our fitness.

The goal of this book is to provide you with the tools and strategies that will empower you to find your own answers to reach higher levels of fitness. But before you can rely on yourself for these answers, you've got to accept full accountability for your successes and failures. If you miss a workout, or gain five pounds, it's not the fault of your boss, your wife, or the weather. It's yours.

You make choices every day that determine your fitness. I have not once heard a champion athlete blame someone or something for lackluster results. Top athletes bring it back to themselves, which empowers them to avoid the same mistake again. That is the frame of mind of champions. Focus on making the necessary changes in your life instead of on blaming others and you will begin to perform at a much higher level.

99. Make Fitness a Family Affair

My dad is the "World's Best Dad." He truly is. I did my first-ever triathlon on St. Croix in the U.S. Virgin Islands. Of course, Dad was there. He always is.

In the triathlon, the key is to move among the three sports—swimming, cycling, and running—with the most possible speed and grace. During the bike portion of the event, I developed stomach cramps—my body wasn't exactly welcoming this new sport. I entered the bike-to-run transition area in second place, my dad practically vibrating with excitement. As I dismounted the bike to head out onto the 10k run, Dad wanted to be sure his boy had enough fuel. So he ran alongside me for the first three hundred meters . . . trying to hand me a glass gallon jug of apple juice and a super-size Butterfinger candy bar. Those of you who race know how unappetizing and impractical those two things are during competition. Realizing this, we both stopped and laughed right there in the middle of one of the toughest events of my life. I remember this moment more than any win.

The point of this story is to encourage you to get your family involved with your fitness. Sharing time during exercise or at athletic events invariably creates richly rewarding memories.

Getting family support for your quest for higher fitness is one of the most important things you can do to ensure long-term success. I would never have made it to my first professional triathlon had it not been for the mind-boggling sacrifices my mother made to buy me the equipment, hire the coaches, and pay for the travel. She is the single reason I became a professional athlete. Similarly, if your wife or husband is truly emotionally behind your efforts, you will exercise more and with more passion.

ACTION ITEM

Schedule a weekly or monthly family workout into your daily planner right now. That workout can be as simple as golfing with your father or hiking with Mom. It's important to get our parents involved in our fitness routines. It maintains a strong bond and keeps them feeling and looking younger.

100. Pass On Your Passion

If there is light in the soul, then there will be beauty in the person. If there is beauty in the person, then there will be harmony in the house. If there is harmony in the house, then there will be order in the nation. And if there is order in the nation, there will be peace in the world.

—CHINESE PROVERB

The power and depth of your passion for exercise will lead to higher performance in your fitness and in your life. I hope this book has provided you with the tools you need to keep the passion afire in your workouts. Building a stronger, healthier body is a powerful thing, but it is ephemeral. What will endure from this will be your self-esteem and your passion for living.

Passion is as infectious as it is powerful. Just as it can transform your life, it can change the lives of people around you.

Take what has touched you most deeply from this book and pass it on to people you care about most. Your passion can inspire and motivate others to change their fitness and their lives in profound ways. And there is no better gift than that.

I wish you all the best.

Appendix A: Ideal Week of Exercise (Five Hours)

Monday: Rest

Tuesday: One-hour key aerobic session (intense)

Wednesday: Thirty-minute strength session

Thursday: Rest

Friday: One-hour aerobic session

Saturday: Two-hour key aerobic session (long)

Sunday: Thirty-minute strength session

To receive personalized Web-based coaching, visit ericharr.com.

Appendix B: The Glycemic Index of Common Foods

The glycemic index is a ranking of foods based on their immediate effect on blood glucose levels. The higher the number, the faster that food elevates blood sugar, which has a deleterious effect on your energy levels and weight-management goals. It has been shown that when your blood sugar levels are constant, you will enjoy steadier energy levels, and your body will more readily metabolize body fat.

Generally, carbohydrates and sugars are higher on the index, while proteins and quality fats are lower. For health, energy, and weight loss, stick to foods lower on the glycemic index (those that fall within the 30–70 range). The numbers listed here are percentages with respect to a reference food, in this case to white bread, which is the standard "reference food" when calculating the glycemic index in the United States.

BAKED GOODS

Muffins	88
Rice cakes	123

BREADS

Barley kernel	49
Rye kernel	71
White bread	101

BREAKFAST CEREALS

All-Bran	60
Cornflakes	119
Oatmeal (non-instant)	87
Shredded wheat	99

FRUIT

Apple	52
Apple juice	58
Banana, overripe	82
Banana, underripe	51
Banana	83
Orange	62
Orange juice	74

GRAINS

Pearl barley	36
Couscous	93
Sweet corn	78
Rice, white	81
Rice, brown	79
Rice, instant	128

DAIRY PRODUCTS

Yogurt, artificially sweetened	27
Milk, whole	39
Milk, skim	46
Ice cream	84

LEGUMES

Kidney beans	42
Kidney beans, canned	74
Lima beans	46
Pinto beans	61
Baked beans	69

PASTA

Spaghetti, non–whole wheat	59
Macaroni	64
Macaroni, boxed	92
Linguine	71

POTATOES

Russet, boiled	80
Russet, mashed	100
Baked	121
French fries	107

SNACKS

Peanuts	21
Popcorn	79
Chocolate (various)	84
Jelly beans	114

SOUPS

Tomato	54
Bean soups (various)	84

SUGARS

Fructose	32
Sucrose (table sugar)	87
Honey	104

Appendix C: World-Class Shopping List

Fresh fish
Lean free-range
   chicken
Muesli
Oats
Bread
Pancake mix
Sugar-free peanut
   butter
Mixed nuts
Cage-free eggs
Tofu
Tuna

Soups/beans
Pasta/rice
Grapefruit
Lemons
Oranges
Grapes
Extra-virgin olive oil
Spinach
Carrots
Celery
Apples
Parsley
Bananas

Squash
Shiitake mushrooms
Tomatoes
Ginger
Red peppers
Garlic

About the Author

Eric Harr is a world-class triathlete, with more than twenty triathlon victories around the world. A California native, he writes the fitness column for the *Marin Independent Journal* and appears on the weekly show *Fitness Friday* on KFTY-50. He is the CEO of Eric Harr Omnimedia, a fitness company. He is the host of a thirteen-part documentary series with Olympic swimmer Dara Torres in which they train with the world's best athletes and learn their innermost wisdom on fitness. He is married and lives and trains in Marin County, California.

I'd love to hear your favorite fitness tips that have created more passion and performance in your life. I may include yours in my next book! Please send to:

Eric Harr
c/o Broadway Books
1540 Broadway, 15th floor
New York, NY 10036

or visit www.ericharr.com.